MW00331988

Practical Child and Adolescent Psychiatry
for Pediatrics and Primary Care

# Endorsements of the Book

Pediatricians and other primary care providers are increasingly being asked to deal with psychological and behavioral problems in their patients. For many of us, our training in these areas was simply not adequate. Along comes a book *Practical Child and Adolescent Psychiatry for Pediatrics and Primary Care* that helps the primary care physician effectively handle these concerns. The authors clearly know the psychiatric issues facing physicians in primary care pediatrics. Their case examples are excellent. As I read many of them, I thought, "I talked to a parent about this just last week!" As the book's title claims, it is very practical. Included are helpful algorithms and diagnostic criteria for many common psychiatric issues facing primary care physicians. Brief summaries of psychotropic medications are just what a primary care physician needs to determine the uses of different medications, as well as their risks and side effects. Their "Clinical Pearls" for many of the medications will be especially helpful. Good information is also available for those medications not commonly prescribed by primary care physicians. This up-to-date handbook will be a valuable resource for pediatricians and other primary care practitioners to effectively diagnose and manage their patients' behavioral problems, and to decide when to refer to a child and adolescent psychiatrist.

*Rickey L. Williams, MD, MPH, President of Tanque Verde Pediatrics, Tucson, AZ*

This is a terrific book, surpassing its promise of providing pediatricians and PCP's with a guide to assessing and treating children and adolescents with mental health problems. Using a remarkably innovative format including descriptions, tables, algorithms and clinical pearls, this format guides clinicians through the challenges of clinical diagnosis, clinical decision-making and treatment. Borrowing from advances in Information Technology and Continuous Quality Improvement processes, the book channels the clinician to pertinent standardized evaluations, symptom and severity checklists, diagnostic criteria and medication recommendations located elsewhere in the book with an ease that approaches a drop down menu and a point and click experience. *Practical Child and Adolescent Psychiatry for Pediatrics and Primary Care* is an exceedingly valuable contribution to the mental health treatment of children and families and the pediatricians and PCP's who will bear much of the responsibility for addressing their needs because of the severe limitations in access to care in the current health care marketplace.

*Robert K. Schreter, MD, Associate Professor of Psychiatry, University of Maryland School of Medicine, Baltimore, MD*

I would predict that the pages of this important book will become worn with daily use by pediatric primary care clinicians in their efforts to care for children with mental health needs. Drs. Trivedi, Kershner, and their colleagues are to be commended for this excellent contribution to the growing field of collaborative child and adolescent psychiatry.

*Barry Sarvet, MD, Massachusetts Child Psychiatry Access Project, Springfield, MA*

Drs. Trivedi and Kershner have given clinicians providing primary care for children and adolescents a valuable tool for approaching the behavioral and psychosocial problems that make up fully one fifth of our practices. Their *Practical Child and Adolescent Psychiatry for Pediatrics and Primary Care* contains resources for diagnosis and management presented in a manner highly relevant to primary care practice. They offer algorithms to approach a child's or adolescent's presenting problem that are clinically relevant and consistent with current practice. Treatment options discussed are relevant to the primary care setting,

recognizing that referral to a mental health professional might not always be timely or even available. This text is likely to become part of the essential library for the primary care office.

*Joseph F. Hagan, Jr., MD, FAAP, Clinical Professor in Pediatrics, University of Vermont College of Medicine, Primary Care Pediatrics, Burlington, VT*

It is increasingly clear that the majority of psychiatric problems will be treated in primary care or pediatric practice. This marvelous volume by a distinguished child psychiatrist and a distinguished pediatrician addresses the growing need to have straightforward practical solution-focused actions that pediatricians and others in primary care practice with children can adopt to deal effectively with common mental health problems in children. The organization of the volume is thoughtful and designed to be quickly and effectively utilized when mental health problems present. The first section describes common chief complaints that typically present in primary care or pediatric practice such as excessive worries or out of control behavior. The second discusses common psychiatric diagnoses and the third, perhaps most importantly, describes what kind of practical actions can be taken for each of these conditions. In fact, intervention toolboxes are provided for each the major conditions and diagnoses. This is an eminently readable, carefully constructed volume and I highly recommend it.

*William R. Beardslee, MD, Academic Chair, Department of Psychiatry, Children's Hospital Boston, MA*

Doctors Trivedi and Kershner have put together an innovative volume that goes well beyond simply providing practical pointers for managing common child and adolescent mental health presentations in primary care settings. Their book is in fact an overarching algorithm that will help non-specialists move out of their erstwhile comfort zones and squarely into the psychiatric domain. With Trivedi and Kershner's guidance, practitioners should expect real results: their clinics will run more smoothly, their consultation requests be fewer and better targeted, and most importantly, the mental health of youths under their care will be addressed in time, on site, and by the very clinicians who know them best.

*Andrés Martin, MD, MPH, Professor of Child Psychiatry and Psychiatry, Director of Medical Studies, Yale Child Study Center and Medical Director of Children's Psychiatric Inpatient Service, Yale-New Haven Children's Hospital, New Haven, CT*

This is a terrific book and resource to both primary care and mental health clinicians. One of the major and common challenges consultants to primary care face is their ability to communicate effectively. Drs Trivedi and Kershner were very successful in using language that is user friendly and well known to primary care clinicians. The use of algorithms throughout the book makes it efficient and fun. Truly great work.

*Lourival Baptista Neto, MD, Director of Clinical Services, Morgan Stanley Children's Hospital of NY Presbyterian/Columbia*

Challenges to mental health are common in children, yet child mental health specialists are scarce. Primary care pediatricians are often the first to face these problems, and must provide much of the treatment even when they feel their training has not fully prepared them to do so. This easy-to-use volume offers practical approaches to screening, assessing and treating the wide range of childhood behavioral and emotional challenges that are carefully adapted to the everyday realities of busy pediatricians. Clear and compassionate, this impressive guide is bound to become a favorite for child mental health specialists as well.

*Joshua Sparrow, MD, Harvard Medical School, Children's Hospital Boston, MA*

# Notice

Child and adolescent psychiatry, like all of medicine, is constantly in flux as new research is published and advancements are made in the field. The authors and the publisher have made every effort to ensure that all information contained in this text is accurate and consistent with current recommendations and generally accepted practice at the time of publication. However, due to changing government regulations, continuing research, and changing information concerning drug therapy and reactions, the reader is urged to check the package insert for any change in indications and dosage, or other added precautions. The authors and publisher disclaim any responsibility for any consequences which may follow from the use of information presented in this book

It is important to note that there are sections of this book for which evidence-based data are not available or where treatments are recommended which are considered "off-label." The authors have attempted to take a conservative perspective when recommending an approach to evaluation and treatment in order to allow for safe and judicious patient care based upon the knowledge base at the time of publication. Application of this material to patient care and ascertainment of current Food and Drug Administration (FDA) status when planning interventions remains the professional responsibility of the practicing physician.

Although the format of the text is algorithmic in nature, it is important to note that this text is not a substitute for a medical examination or consultation with a physician. Please note that due to the individual needs of specific patients, or due to certain clinical situations, appropriate clinical care may require assessment, treatment, and monitoring different from what is covered in this text. Consultation with a physician specialist, such as a child and adolescent psychiatrist, should be considered for recommendations regarding specific patients that you are treating. Readers are encouraged to verify the information presented in this text with current information in other sources.

Nonphysicians, lay readers, regulators, courts, or legislative bodies should note that significant portions of information for the safe evaluation and management of patients are not presented in this text as they are an integral part of medical training for physicians. The algorithms in this text are not a substitute for sound medical judgment. They should not be applied by practitioners without a medical degree, appropriate Accreditation Council for Graduate Medical Education (ACGME) certified residency or fellowship training, and current active medical licensure. All questions about treatments or therapies should be directed to a physician.

## Conflict of Interest Statement / Disclosures

Dr. Trivedi and Dr. Kershner have made all efforts to ensure that the information presented in this text is free of bias. They do not have any conflicts of interest to disclose. They do not receive any compensation nor do they have any other such relationships with pharmaceutical companies or medical device manufacturers.

**Library of Congress Cataloging in Publication**

is available via the Library of Congress Marc Database under the
LC Control Number 2008939655

**Library and Archives Canada Cataloguing in Publication**

Trivedi, Harsh K.
    Practical child and adolescent psychiatry for pediatrics and primary care / Harsh K.
Trivedi, Jeryl Dansky Kershner.

Includes bibliographical references.
ISBN 978-0-88937-349-5
1. Child psychiatry--Handbooks, manuals, etc. 2. Adolescent psychiatry--Handbooks,
manuals, etc. I. Kershner, Jeryl Dansky II. Title.

RJ499.3.T75 2008          618.92'89          C2008-905885-2


© 2009 by Hogrefe & Huber Publishers

PUBLISHING OFFICES
USA:            Hogrefe & Huber Publishers, 875 Massachusetts Avenue, 7th Floor,
                Cambridge, MA 02139
                Phone (866) 823-4726, Fax (617) 354-6875; E-mail info@hogrefe.com
EUROPE:         Hogrefe & Huber Publishers, Rohnsweg 25, 37085 Göttingen, Germany
                Phone +49 551 49609-0, Fax +49 551 49609-88, E-mail hh@hogrefe.com

SALES & DISTRIBUTION
USA:            Hogrefe & Huber Publishers, Customer Services Department,
                30 Amberwood Parkway, Ashland, OH 44805
                Phone (800) 228-3749, Fax (419) 281-6883, E-mail custserv@hogrefe.com
EUROPE:         Hogrefe & Huber Publishers, Rohnsweg 25, 37085 Göttingen, Germany
                Phone +49 551 49609-0, Fax +49 551 49609-88, E-mail hh@hogrefe.com

OTHER OFFICES
CANADA:         Hogrefe & Huber Publishers, 1543 Bayview Avenue, Toronto, Ontario M4G 3B5
SWITZERLAND:    Hogrefe & Huber Publishers, Länggass-Strasse 76, CH-3000 Bern 9

Hogrefe & Huber Publishers
Incorporated and registered in the State of Washington, USA, and in Göttingen, Lower Saxony, Germany

Printed and bound in the USA
ISBN: 978-0-88937-349-5

# Practical Child and Adolescent Psychiatry
## for Pediatrics and Primary Care

**Harsh K. Trivedi, MD**

Diplomate, American Board of Psychiatry & Neurology
Subspecialty Certification in Child & Adolescent Psychiatry
Site Training Director & Director of Adolescent Services, Bradley Hospital, Providence, RI
Assistant Professor of Psychiatry and Human Behavior (Clinical), Brown Alpert Medical School, Providence, RI
Consulting Editor, *Child & Adolescent Psychiatric Clinics of North America*
President, Rhode Island Council of Child and Adolescent Psychiatry, Providence, RI

**Jeryl Dansky Kershner, MD, FAAP**

Diplomate, American Board of Pediatrics
Subspecialty Certification in Developmental Behavioral Pediatrics
Fellowship Trained in Child and Adolescent Psychiatry, Children's Hospital Boston
Alpert Jewish Family and Children's Services, West Palm Beach, FL

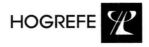

# Dedication

To those who taught me compassion, humanity, and work ethic –
*Balashankar P. Trivedi, Markand G. Rawal, & Ramesh J. Trivedi*

To those who sustain me and propel me to strive onward –
*Kirit, Pratima, Maulik, Mala, Dylan, Sonya, family, & friends*

To those who allow me into their lives to help them –
*the youth, parents, and families I work with daily*

And to the one who means everything to me –
*my wife, Urmi*

HKT

To my husband Robert,
*who continues to open doors and has encouraged me to follow my dreams*

To my two daughters, Shaina and Emily,
*who have taught me that parenting is a great challenge,
a humbling experience, and the most rewarding job in the world*

To the families
*who have allowed me the privilege of being a part of their lives*

JDK

# Foreword

In the realm of child mental health services, pediatricians and primary care providers are often unsung heroes. When there is limited access to mental health professionals, when stigma associated with psychiatrists or psychologists makes parents hesitant to use them, or when the vagaries of managed care preclude referrals to specific mental health professionals, you are the ones being asked to fill the void. Most often this is done, though, with varying degrees of enthusiasm.

Our medical system certainly doesn't make it easy for primary care physicians to be mental health providers. Reimbursement is a significant problem, as arcane rules make it difficult, for example, for a pediatrician to get paid when billing for "depression" as opposed to a "urinary tract infection." Too often it seems that society's expectation is for a primary care physician to provide psychiatric services in *less* time than it takes me to do the job – even though I have had more training and many years of experience treating psychiatric problems.

In my experience, however, the financial hardship is not the main factor behind primary care physicians' hesitancy – when it occurs – to deal with children's mental health issues. Much more salient is the concern about their expertise in the mental health arena. I've frequently heard variations on the following:

> "There are so many controversies in child psychiatry and the field is changing so fast that it seems like a minefield – so much to know."

> "My residency training was light in the behavioral realm – I don't feel competent."

or

> "Child psychiatry isn't my main interest – I'm afraid I don't read enough to be up-to-date."

I certainly resonate with those sentiments: truth be told, I'm not that enthusiastic about evaluating a 6-year-old's earache or a teenager's belly pain when it's my turn to be the weekend attending on our inpatient psychiatric units. The difference is that I have immediate access to pediatric consultation and can refer the patient at will. Rarely do primary care physicians have the same options when it comes to their patients' psychiatric problems. Hence, the heroism.

This book represents a big step forward as it provides high-quality, practical psychiatric information in an accessible form for busy pediatricians and primary care providers. Dr. Trivedi, Dr. Kershner, and their collaborators have combined their extensive knowledge of child and adolescent psychiatry with an awareness of the realities of primary care to produce a gem of a resource book. It is extremely up-to-date, without getting mired in the latest debates about forms of bipolar disorder or how one should prescribe antipsychotics to 2-year-olds. The book is – as it should be – balanced between psychosocial and biological approaches. It is appropriately without influence from the pharmaceutical industry.

My sense is that with a reference like this at your fingertips you will be more competent, confident, and comfortable in your role as a child mental health provider. When that happens, children will be the true beneficiaries.

Gregory K. Fritz, MD

Professor and Director
Division of Child and Adolescent Psychiatry
Department of Psychiatry and Human Behavior
Brown Alpert Medical School

Academic Director
Bradley Hospital

Associate Chief and Director of Child Psychiatry
Rhode Island Hospital and
Hasbro Children's Hospital

# Preface

If you have picked up this book, you are likely all too aware of the staggering problems that exist both in the prevalence of child and adolescent mental illnesses as well as in finding trained specialists to care for them.

## The Problem

The US Surgeon General estimates that one out of five children and adolescents between the ages of nine and seventeen has a diagnosable mental or addictive disorder causing functional impairment. Within the United States alone, this equates to over 10 million youths that require mental health treatment. It is estimated that it would take 30,000 child and adolescent psychiatrists to meet this need. Unfortunately, less than one fourth of that number, only about 7,000, are currently in practice.

As Dr. Thomas F. Anders, a past president of the American Academy of Child and Adolescent Psychiatry, put it "There is a serious crisis in the child and adolescent psychiatry workforce. There are far too few of us, and large parts of the country – especially rural and inner city areas – have few, if any, child and adolescent psychiatrists… Fewer than half of the children in need of care are evaluated, and even fewer are treated effectively." Due to the severe shortage of child and adolescent psychiatrists, the vast majority of these patients are seen by pediatricians and other primary care providers (PCPs) for the diagnosis and treatment of their mental health problems.

## Two Paths: One Goal

It isn't completely random that of all the people who might write a book on this topic, Jeryl Kershner and I were the ones who felt compelled to make it happen. We first met during our child and adolescent psychiatry fellowship at Children's Hospital Boston. She was a seasoned pediatrician with over twenty years of experience. In her pediatric practice, she had been treating kids with mental health problems for years now; so much so that she was commonly referred patients from her pediatric colleagues. She had a growing frustration about how these patients got (or didn't get) the help they needed. She decided to go back for additional training and joined the Developmental Behavioral Pediatrics Fellowship at Children's Hospital Boston. Wanting to know more, she boldly decided to do what would most help her patients. She left her pediatric comfort zone in order to pursue child and adolescent psychiatry fellowship training.

I had quite a different professional path to arrive at the same training program. I had fallen in love with pediatrics during medical school at Mount Sinai. I had seriously considered joining their "Triple Board Program" (combined 5 year training in pediatrics, psychiatry, and child and adolescent psychiatry), but in the end knew that my true calling was to go where I was most needed (child and adolescent psychiatry). After completing my general psychiatry training, I was selected as a congressional fellow and was placed in the Washington, DC office of Senator Jack Reed (D-RI). I had the fortune of helping to develop language for one of the few pieces of mental health legislation that got enacted during that time. The Garrett Lee Smith Memorial Act provided funding (over $80 million over 3 years) for developing suicide prevention programs and improving college mental health services nationally. I quickly learned about the difference I could make by working for larger systemic changes. Indeed my work as a congressional fellow allowed me to accomplish more with the stroke of a pen and help far more people than I can ever hope to treat as a physician diligently working with my patients over a thirty-plus year career. As I was entering the child and adolescent psychiatry fellowship at Children's Hospital Boston, I had a renewed sense of direction – to not only hone my clinical skills, but to also keep my eyes open for the next opportunity to improve the lives of children and families affected by mental illness.

Despite our very different professional paths, Dr. Kershner and I share one thing: At the heart of our professional passion is an earnest desire to fundamentally improve the lives those we treat daily.

## A Common Understanding

We both recognized that most pediatricians and PCPs have little exposure to the routine assessment and treatment of mental or addictive disorders during training. Despite a lack of appropriate training or clinical expertise, they are routinely confronted with the difficult task of having to triage, differentially diagnose, and treat many of these issues.

Imagine going through your entire residency training and never really being taught about how to listen for lung sounds, about how to diagnose and treat respiratory ailments, or about the appropriate management of RSV or asthma. Now imagine starting your first job in the dead of winter, during flu season, and 20% of the patients walking through your door are complaining of difficulty breathing, shortness of breath, or wheezing. You would likely get a gnawing feeling in your stomach that you were inadequately prepared to help a large number of your patients.

Unfortunately, a similar event already occurs daily when that same patient walks through the door with a mental health problem. Without really being taught about how to diagnose and treat basic psychiatric conditions, 20% of the patients in your practice may need help for mental health conditions as common and as basic as RSV or asthma. Now you may *really* have that gnawing feeling recur, but this time it is with good reason.

## So Many Obstacles

As if all of this wasn't enough, the recent Food and Drug Administration black box warning for stimulants and antidepressants has only created further anxiety amongst providers in helping to care for this population. Add to that the recent announcement and retraction from the American Heart Association that all kids starting stimulants need an electrocardiogram. When combining all of these pressures with the fact that most pediatricians and PCPs see 40–60 patients per day, the obvious question is: How can you take care of the most common psychiatric presentations that walk through your door every day? How can you do it while ensuring quality mental health care? Not to mention, how can you do this, while continuing to meet the needs of all the other patients that you see daily?

For the physicians reading this preface, there is some part of you that resonates with this frustration. You have patients who certainly are having problems, but you aren't sure what they are. Even if you do remember from your medical school rotation that you are seeing the signs of depression, what is the current standard of care? How do you evaluate the severity of the symptoms? How do you determine what type of treatment the patient needs? And just as important, how do you manage to take care of this patient in the midst of a busy practice without falling two hours behind?

You do not have the time to read reference texts or to extensively research the current literature between patients. What you need is a book that is easily accessible, practical, and useful, and that places clinically relevant information at your fingertips.

## The Solution

Combining our knowledge and professional experience, we quickly realized that we were in a unique situation to understand both the needs of pediatricians and PCPs, while also understanding the needs of the patients who present to a child and adolescent psychiatrist for the treatment of their mental health problems. We spoke to many colleagues and families about what would be most helpful – and how we could help the most kids get needed access to quality competent care. We heard from many people who passionately spoke about the need for this book, a different kind of handbook, one that gave only the information that would be most helpful to you: A book that is written specifically for a pediatric and PCP audience, not getting bogged down with too much psychiatry, and having clear algorithmic steps of what to do.

As opposed to chapters on psychiatric diagnoses (which aren't so helpful if you don't know what the diagnosis is), we start with the chief complaints that you are likely to encounter. We provide algorithms to guide you through the assessment and treatment of children and adolescents with mental health problems. Our hope is that this structure will help you to develop a framework in your own mind to think about these issues. We then allow you to input your clinical judgment to determine what the next steps are and subsequently lead you through progressive parts of the book to the key information that you need:

– Did you ever wonder whether your patient should get a trial of therapy before starting medications? We help you figure that out.
– Did you ever wonder which medicine to start, at what dose, how to titrate, what to tell parents, and how to manage it? We help you with that as well.
– Did you ever ask yourself which rating scale would be helpful in monitoring a child's progress?

Done.

## The Goal

We want you to feel just as comfortable treating a child with ADHD, depression, or separation anxiety disorder as you would treating a child with an ear infection, the flu, or asthma. We know that you

want to provide conscientious and competent care. We know that you want tips on how to structure your practice so that it can function smoothly even when a psychiatrically urgent or emergent patient is seen.

In creating this book, we have made every effort to best address your needs. As you read through it yourself, we also need your help. We welcome your feedback so that we can make future editions even more useful. Most importantly, we sincerely hope that the book will provide you with the tools to better help your patients. Thank you.

Harsh K. Trivedi
(harsh_trivedi@brown.edu)

Jeryl Dansky Kershner
(drkershner@mykidspsych.com)

## References

Anders TF (2008) Child and Adolescent Psychiatry: The Next Ten Years. *Psychiatric Times,* 2008;25(6).

Kim WJ, Enzer N, Bechtold D, et al. Meeting the Mental Health Needs of Children and Adolescents: Addressing the Problems of Access to Care. Report of the Task Force on Workforce Needs. Washington, DC: American Academy of Child and Adolescent Psychiatry; 2001.

US Department of Health and Human Services. *Mental Health: A Report of the Surgeon General.* Rockville, MD: US Dept of Health and Human Services; 1999.

# Contributors

The following contributors aided in the research and writing of this text. In creating the innovative format for this book, we acknowledge and thank them for agreeing to have their "traditional" chapters broken down and reconstructed to mesh into the algorithmic format presented. This has required much flexibility on their part and an earnest willingness to allow for significant rewriting of their work. Indeed, most chapters are an amalgam of multiple contributors. The contributors are listed below based upon the chief complaint or topic area that they worked on. Please note that they have also contributed to subsequent diagnosis and treatment sections based upon where their chief complaint or topic areas mapped onto the algorithms. This has allowed for the creation of a clearly written, well designed, practical, and useful text. It is our hope that this book will help many youths get needed access to quality care.

Amy E. Cousineau, MSW, LICSW
*Psychotherapeutic and Psychosocial Interventions*
Social Worker, Adolescent Program
Bradley Hospital

Emily Katz, MD, FAAP
*Sudden Personality Change or Confusion*
Chief Resident, Child and Adolescent Psychiatry
Assistant Instructor
Dept. of Psychiatry and Human Behavior
Brown Alpert Medical School

Elizabeth D. Kowal, MD
*Excessive Worries*
Resident, Triple Board Program
Combined Program in Pediatrics, Psychiatry, &
    Child Psychiatry
Brown Alpert Medical School

Gina M. Liguori, BS
*Suggested Rating Scales*
Psychology Assistant
Bradley Hospital

Elizabeth A. Lowenhaupt, MD, FAAP
*Fatigue or Changes in Appetite*
Assistant Professor
Dept. of Psychiatry and Human Behavior
Brown Alpert Medical School

Lisa Maccarone Goldstein, MSW, LICSW
*Psychotherapeutic and Psychosocial Interventions*
Social Worker, Adolescent Program
Bradley Hospital

Gary R. Maslow, MD
*Recurrent Mild Medical Complaints*
Resident, Triple Board Program
Combined Program in Pediatrics, Psychiatry, &
    Child Psychiatry
Assistant Instructor
Dept. of Psychiatry and Human Behavior
Brown Alpert Medical School

Tracy K. Mullare, MD
*Irritable or Out-of-Control Behavior*
Chief Resident, Triple Board Program
Combined Program in Pediatrics, Psychiatry, &
    Child Psychiatry
Assistant Instructor
Dept. of Psychiatry and Human Behavior
Brown Alpert Medical School

Sherri Sharp, MD
*School Refusal*
Resident, Child and Adolescent Psychiatry
Assistant Instructor
Dept. of Psychiatry and Human Behavior
Brown Alpert Medical School

Matthew Siegel, MD
*Speech Problems or Refusing to Speak*
Chief Resident, Triple Board Program
Combined Program in Pediatrics, Psychiatry, &
    Child Psychiatry
Assistant Instructor
Dept. of Psychiatry and Human Behavior
Brown Alpert Medical School

# Acknowledgements

The authors give special thanks to our wonderful publisher, Robert Dimbleby, and his team at Hogrefe and Huber for their help and expertise in seeing this project to completion. We appreciate the support and guidance given by everyone at Bradley Hospital (especially Dan Wall, Dr. Henry Sachs III, Dr. Jeffrey I. Hunt, and Ann Beardsley) – a place where we *do* heal the hearts and minds of kids and their families every day. Likewise, we are grateful to Dr. Gregory K. Fritz, Division Chair of Child and Adolescent Psychiatry, and the Department of Psychiatry and Human Behavior at the Brown Alpert Medical School for their ongoing support. We wish to thank our professional medical organizations for being actively engaged in helping youth and their families obtain access to quality and competent care. In particular, we thank our colleagues and supporters at the American Academy of Child and Adolescent Psychiatry, the American Academy of Pediatrics, the American Psychiatric Association, and the American Medical Association. Most importantly, the impetus for creating this book as well as for believing that fundamental change can occur for the common good was instilled by working in the office of Senator Jack Reed (D-RI). We are thankful to the Senator and his entire staff (particularly Neil Campbell, Lisa German-Foster, and Rosanne Haroian) for their support and ongoing guidance. The entire Rhode Island Congressional delegation is one that must be applauded for not only its steadfast support but also its key leadership on issues that matter to children and their families. Special thanks in this regard go to Congressman Patrick J. Kennedy (D-RI) for his work on the Child Health Care Crisis Relief Act. We also thank Missy Tatum for her help in the preparation of this manuscript.

# Table of Contents

# List of Algorithms

# Section I
# Getting Ready

This section presents information related to planning for the evaluation and treatment of youth with mental illness.

It will cover the following topics:

- How to Use This Book
- Setting Up Your Office

# 1 How to Use This Book

Not too many medical texts you purchase will come with instructions. Then again, not many medical texts have devoted as much thought and energy to creating an educational aide as we have for this one. Our goal is to not only provide you with a fund of knowledge about child and adolescent psychiatry, but hopefully, to also help you in developing a thought process to think like a child and adolescent psychiatrist. When evaluating children and adolescents with mental health issues in your office, we want you to not only pick the best course of action but to also truly understand the method by which that clinical decision was made. This in itself is a large task, one that usually requires a 2-year fellowship, after 3 or 4 years of general psychiatry training, plus at least another handful of years in practice to get it right. Although we may not make you into a child and adolescent psychiatrist, we do want to help you understand the rationale behind thoughtful assessment and treatment.

Each section is designed to help you in developing this framework. We introduce a step-by-step methodology so that you can learn a safe and comprehensive approach to differential diagnosis, assessment, and treatment. This is written as a programmed text in that it leads you through each successive step of the evaluation by allowing for your clinical input and medical judgment to determine the direction in which to take the case. As you work through this format and start understanding the thought process, you will find that you will need to reference earlier parts of this book less and less. By allowing your own clinical impressions to guide you through this text, we help you to engrain certain automatic responses. For example, if a patient states that he has had recent fleeting suicidal thoughts, we refer you to the Appendix to learn how to conduct a comprehensive safety and risk assessment. As you learn the appropriate questions

to ask, over time, you may find yourself no longer needing to look at that appendix for the "right" questions to ask. By having algorithms that lead you to appropriate portions of the book, we help you to develop your thought process while getting familiar with the knowledge base as well.

As marvelous as this sounds, it is important to note that this format does not allow for the appropriate management of all cases nor all severities of illness. Every effort has been made to address routine presentations of common illnesses. The best analogy would be a generalist and specialist model. If a patient presented to you with malaise, fever, and recent weight loss, you would know how to work up and treat the most common illnesses. As you went down your differential, if you determined that it may be a case of acute lymphoblastic leukemia, you would likely refer out to a specialist.

Similarly for child and adolescent psychiatry, we believe that there is a core of diagnosis and treatment that can be safely assessed and appropriately treated in the primary care office. If there are more complicated cases or cases refractory to your treatment, they should be referred to the specialist. We have thought about the situations where the algorithm goes beyond what most pediatricians and primary care physicians (PCPs) can safely and routinely treat in their office. In these instances, we clearly delineate when to refer to a child and adolescent psychiatrist. We acknowledge that for some advanced practitioners, you may feel that our arbitrary line in the sand for when to refer occurs too soon. Our experience in discussing the referral points with more novice practitioners is that their sentiment was quite the opposite – wanting to consult the specialist sooner. In trying to strike this balance, we have decided upon rational points in treatment where consulting a specialist may be quite helpful. Your decision of when to refer should be guided by your own comfort level and level of expertise.

As such, we understand that there is a wide spectrum of exposure and comfort in dealing with children and adolescent psychiatric issues among pediatricians and primary care physicians (PCPs). In attempting to meet you at your current level of expertise, the book is divided into four sections. For those who are pre-contemplative about whether this can be done in the primary care setting or for those who already do it but want to become more efficient, we offer Section I in the book entitled "Getting Ready." It addresses the main concerns about getting more involved in the assessment and treatment of these common disorders. We walk you through the practicalities of setting up your office, scheduling appointments, optimally using support staff, incorporating the use of rating scales, and more. Once you have reviewed this section, you will likely refer to it only minimally in the course of evaluating patients.

The second section is "Approach to Common Chief Complaints." As opposed to other texts which have "traditional" chapters divided by psychiatric diagnoses, this text starts one step back with chief complaints. Most likely, parents will not come to you and say "I think my child has major depressive disorder, recurrent, severe, with psychotic features. Can you help me?" Based upon Dr. Kershner's years of experience dealing with patients and parents in a pediatric primary care office, we have developed a list of the most common chief complaints that you are likely to encounter. We realize that this is not an exhaustive list of complaints. These particular ones have been chosen because they map onto the main categories of psychiatric disorders and treatments. While working up these chief complaints, you will become facile at thinking through other chief complaints in the process as well.

Another difference from more traditional medical texts is that chapters are usually written by different authors and then edited for content and format. This can lead to books that vary in tone, length, language, and quality from chapter to chapter. We acknowledge the contributors of this text for agreeing to have their traditional chapters broken down and reconstructed to mesh into the algorithmic format presented. This has required much flexibility on their part and an earnest willingness to allow for significant rewriting of their work. Indeed, most chapters are an amalgam of multiple contributors. This has allowed for the creation of a clearly written, well designed, practical, and useful text that is consistent from chapter to chapter.

The feature that you will notice most about the chapters from Section II onwards is that they have limited text and present multiple figures and tables. During the midst of a busy day, we want this to be a ready reference. Indeed, most of the key information that you will likely use over and over again is presented in graphical form as a figure or table. Each chapter is meant to be easily accessible and reviewable within 3–5 minutes. Any longer and this book would likely join the other books on your shelf that you would love to read when you have more time.

In trying to create this balance, there are two important points to keep in mind. The first is that we know that you are a pediatrician or PCP. For this reason, we do not belabor the medical work-up or cover issues that you already know. For example, we do not cover child abuse as a freestanding chapter nor do we tell you to look for fractures at different stages of healing. We know that any appropriately trained pediatrician or PCP is well aware of this. To keep this handbook from becoming unwieldy, we only focus on the information that you may be less familiar with.

Secondly, it is important to keep in mind that we are also limiting the psychiatric information that we present. By limiting ourselves to the key clinical information that applies to most patients and is most relevant to what you can assess and treat in a primary care office, we are able to present information that you can review quickly. For example, we do not walk you through the assessment algorithm for learning disorders or mental retardation. Although they may present, you will not be the one conducting educational, cognitive, psychological, or neurological testing. We would expect that you would refer to a specialist if a concern arose. Please remember that this is not an authoritative textbook; it is meant to be a practical handbook. Our focus is on helping you to provide care. If you need more in-depth information, we have suggested references at the back of the book to guide the user to other well-trusted sources.

Each chief complaint provides *Clinical Snapshots* 📷 of likely presentations, *Key Points* ⚷ describing take home messages for the physician, a *Psychiatric Differential Diagnosis* with an *Assessment Algorithm*, and *Take Home Messages* 🗒 for the patient, parent, and family. Your clinical input will help lead you through the algorithm to relevant portions of the book regarding diagnosis and treatment in subsequent sections. As you become more familiar with the work-up of these chief complaints, you may find yourself referring only to the assessment algorithm or going directly to the diagnosis and treatment sections. As this occurs, you will likely become more efficient and more comfortable with the material.

Section III then presents information related to accurately diagnosing psychiatric illnesses and determining severity of symptoms. Each chapter provides an *Assessment Algorithm* based upon DSM-IV-TR®[1] and a *Severity Assessment and Treatment Algorithm* to determine the level of intervention required. Levels of severity are divided into routine, urgent, and emergent. Your clinical input will help lead you through the algorithm to relevant portions of the book regarding the treatment options in subsequent sections. As you become more familiar with these diagnoses, you may find yourself referring only to the diagnostic algorithm or going directly to the treatment section.

Section IV presents information related to treatment options for psychiatric illnesses. The treatments are subdivided into biological interventions, psychotherapeutic interventions, and psychosocial interventions. Each chapter provides a *Treatment Description* and *Clinical Pearls* to maximize treatment efficacy while limiting potential side effects. As you become more familiar with these treatments, you may find yourself *significantly impacting the lives of the children and adolescents you treat*. Hence, as we first asserted: This is not your average medical text.

---

[1]    DSM-IV-TR® is a trademark of the American Psychiatric Association.

# 2 Setting Up Your Office

In talking to pediatricians and PCPs about their greatest concerns with providing mental health assessment and treatment in their practices, a number of practical issues recurrently came up, such as optimizing practice structure, utilizing support staff, and managing kids and families in crisis. This chapter was written to address many of those concerns, which are likely similar to the concerns that you have as well.

We understand that pediatric and primary care practices have significant variation in regards to location of the practice, number of providers, patient population served, support staff present, availability of child and adolescent mental health service providers, and a multitude of other characteristics. In attempting to distill the most important suggestions for setting up your office, the following general suggestions were selected as those that would be effective in a majority of practice settings with minimal need to drastically change office functions. Further specification of these recommendations to meet your practice's individual needs is suggested as the applicability and implementation of these steps will vary from practice to practice.

## Start with What You've Got

Before trying to figure out everything that you need to change, take two steps back and conduct a needs assessment. It is important to first figure out what things you already do well and what areas require further attention. Ask your staff as well as your patients and their parents about how you could improve things. Let them know that you are considering some changes to better improve mental health care in the office and get their thoughts about what they would like to see. This will help you to prioritize where you should devote initial

energies. As a part of this discussion, let them know to expect that some hiccups may occur and that you want them to tell you when they happen. Reassure them you are committed to helping them and that you will be responsive to the concerns that are raised.

## Comprehensive Solutions Require a Team

Your office is probably a busy place filled with kids ranging in age from newborns to college-bound young adults. You probably rush from patient to patient, taking care of runny noses, sprained ankles, belly pains, and a host of other chief complaints. You likely field urgent phone calls from concerned parents as well as respond to calls from other providers and consultants. You probably have some days when you go about doing one thing after the other, not even realizing where the time went. Somewhere in the midst of this controlled chaos exists the glue that keeps many practices going. As we paint this all too familiar picture, the truth is that having great support staff can make all the difference with how well your practice functions on a day to day basis.

In order to appropriately assess, treat, and manage youth mental health issues in your practice, you will need to have support staff who are well trained, who know how to respond, and are aware of their role in this process. Just as you may have concerns about how this will practically occur in the midst of your practice, they too will have their concerns. Before enacting the changes that we recommend below, we ask you to gauge your staff's level of anxiety as well as their willingness or buy-in to caring for youth with mental health problems in the office.

Make sure that staff members have an avenue for voicing their questions and concerns to you or the practice administrator. As you start implementing changes to optimize your practice procedures, there needs to be an on-going opportunity for receiving their feedback and for adjusting office processes to better fit your practice structure. Indeed, they may often catch on to issues long before you become aware of them.

## Setting the Tone for Practice Functions

As much as there is an avenue for open communication, it is important that you set the tone for patient care in the practice. As both you and your staff enter new unfamiliar waters in addressing mental health concerns, it is important that you dictate the level of service and tone for treatment that staff will adopt. There needs to be an expectation, coming from you, that all staff members are ready and willing to support patients and families with mental health issues. It should not be perceived as one more burden in their day, especially by the patient or family.

That being said, the clearer your expectations are, the easier it will be for everyone. In particular, thought should be given about what you can *and cannot* handle in your office. As previously mentioned, each practice and each practitioner may be at different places in their level of comfort with assessing and treating different psychiatric diagnoses. Your staff should understand your level of comfort as well as have an understanding of their own internal barometer. If there are multiple physicians in your practice, it may be easier for your staff if the providers have developed a consistent message of what can and cannot be handled in the office.

A key point to discuss from the beginning is that as your level of comfort increases, the types of cases that you treat may also change. In the best case scenario, your staff will also be progressing in their level of comfort in dealing with mental health issues as well.

## Nothing Decreases Anxiety Like Knowledge and Reassurance

There are probably some staff members that you can already identify in your office who tend to do well with patients and parents in crisis. They may be the ones who are most excited and looking forward to your willingness to start more comprehensive assessment and treatment of mental health problems. Utilize these people as your resources and allow them to get other staff members on the same page. Identify ways that they can be helpful and use their positive energy to create traction in the office. In short, think about all of the ways that you can utilize them more efficiently.

The next main obstacle for most people is lack of knowledge. People tend to be apprehensive of things they are unfamiliar with. Try to figure out how you can schedule an in-service or lunch training with staff to help ease their anxiety. Also, don't assume that you need to cover everything in one session. Just as you don't want to overload parents with too much information, break things down to more manageable pieces and provide the trainings over the course of weeks to months. At the outset, however, if you plan on doing additional sessions in the future, let them know about it.

Another great resource comes in the form of pamphlets created by the professional associations. Both the American Academy of Child and Adolescent Psychiatry's *Facts for Families* (www.aacap.org) and the American Academy of Pediatrics *Guidelines for Parents* (www.aap.org) are valuable handouts to have in your office. Leave copies of these in your lunchroom or break area so staff members can familiarize themselves with the information. They will be learning the information themselves and will then be able to handout appropriate pamphlets to patients and parents. Encourage your staff to review these handouts and to use the information to support and guide patients and families.

Also think of other important pieces of information that would be helpful for them to learn. For example, have an in-service with staff regarding the mental status exam. It will help your staff to monitor for important signs and to better communicate their observations to you. A sample format for the mental status exam is reviewed in Appendix A. Have them practice filling out a sample mental status exam on selected patients and then compare it to your findings.

## Decreasing the Element of Surprise Through Routine Assessment

We have had providers tell us that they don't use routine assessments or try not to ask too many probing questions because they aren't sure what they would do if they did find something. Others have expressed a fear about the level of uncertainty that mental health problems create in their daily schedules and how the rest of their patient care hours take a toll when a psychiatrically urgent or emergent patient must be seen.

Although this may seem counter-intuitive, if you start routinely assessing for mental health issues, you will actually have fewer surprises when a patient is in a crisis. Additionally, as you get better at assessment and treatment, you will also help to avert many of these situations from ever occurring. We recommend that you incorporate the use of a standard general screening questionnaire for all patients at routine intervals. These can be handed out by your receptionist and should be completed in the waiting room. Consider using the Pediatric Symptom Checklist or the Child Behavior Check List (see Appendix E). Once completed, get your support staff to review and score these assessments for you. Have them flag the ones that are of concern for your review.

In addition to the use of a general screening tool, adopt a method of incorporating the use of specific rating scales depending on the chief complaint. If a patient or parent brings up concerning issues regarding depression in the general screening or comes in with a chief complaint of depression, have support staff already trained to give out a depression rating scale. If you are already treating an adolescent for depression, have the patient and parent fill out a depression rating scale at successive visits to monitor progress. Adding these additional steps will add structure

to your practice and provide you with valuable information.

If you get a core group of rating scales together that you and your staff are familiar with, keep them in a central location near your check-in area and get everyone into the habit of utilizing them. An often overlooked point is to also incorporate a uniform location in your chart to file completed scales for future reference and to track scores over time to monitor progress. Rating scales are reviewed in Appendix E. When you get a positive screening, review it with your staff to reinforce not only the importance of the rating scale, but also their role in this process.

## Realistic Scheduling and Improved Triage Can Help to Improve Your Mental Health

Nothing is harder to do during the course of a busy day than to catch up with your schedule. At the outset, let us be clear in stating that patients with mental health problems can not be scheduled the same as every other patient that walks through the door. Expect that you will need to spend more time with them, especially in the beginning. It is best to keep dedicated time for scheduling patients with mental health issues. For example, for routine follow-ups (nonurgent and nonemergent cases) have one afternoon a week set aside for such kids. If you can't schedule out a block of time, try to schedule these appointments with built in buffers. For example, schedule them later in the day or before a charting or lunch break, so that you can spend a little extra time with them if needed, and so that it doesn't throw off the rest of your patient schedule. For those who can incorporate evening hours into your practice, this is also a good time to schedule appointments for mental health concerns. How much time you set aside will be based on how many such patients you regularly see. Expect to schedule at least 30 minutes for an initial visit and approximately 15 minutes for a follow-up appointment.

One of the mistakes that we sometimes see is that the receptionist books patients with mental health issues in the middle of same day urgent appointments. Although they may be urgent, they will definitely take more time than a regular urgent patient. A word to the wise would be to avoid situations that are set up to fail. Help to train your staff about how to figure out with the parent whether the patient falls into the urgent or emergent categories. Any parent who is concerned about the immediate safety of their child or of other family members, hence an emergent case, should be referred to an emergency room. All psychiatric emergencies should be referred to your local emergency room for an emergency psychiatric evaluation. Urgent cases, those that do not need to be seen immediate-ly but do require your attention, should be scheduled to see you within 24–72 hours depending on the presentation. Routine evaluations or follow-up appointments can be scheduled within 3–7 days.

By following these tips, we hope that you will find both you and your staff feeling more comfortable with addressing the mental health concerns of the patients and families that you are caring for. Being open to making adjustments and tailoring our suggestions to fit your practice will lead to the best outcomes. Also, if there are important things that you learn along the way, please let us know so that we can let others know (see contact information in the Preface).

# Section II
# Approach to Common Chief Complaints

This section presents information related to the clinical approach for evaluating common chief complaints. Each chief complaint provides *Clinical Snapshots* of likely presentations, *Key Points* describing take home messages for the physician, a *Psychiatric Differential Diagnosis* with an *Assessment Algorithm*, and *Take Home Messages* for the patient, parent, and family. Your clinical input will help lead you through the algorithm to relevant portions of the book regarding diagnosis and treatment in subsequent sections. As you become more familiar with the work-up of these chief complaints, you may find yourself referring only to the algorithm or going directly to the diagnosis and treatment sections.

It covers the following chief complaints:

- Irritable or Out-of-Control Behavior
- Fatigue or Changes in Appetite
- School Refusal
- Recurrent Mild Medical Complaints
- Speech Problems or Refusing to Speak
- Sudden Personality Change or Confusion
- Excessive Worries

# 3 Irritable Or Out-Of-Control Behavior

## Clinical Snapshots

Christine is a four-year-old girl with no significant past medical history who presents at your office for a well-child visit. Mom explains that she has been more irritable lately and has "not been herself." She tends to be more withdrawn and interacts less with other kids in the neighborhood. She gets tired more easily and is quick to snap at others. She recently pushed another child and has started stomping her feet when she doesn't get her way. Mom states that these behaviors are new for her and that she is usually quite happy and well behaved.

Adam is a 16-year-old boy with a history of asthma. He is a "B"-student and has had some minor behavioral issues in the past. He received detention for silly and disrespectful behavior last year, but is doing better this year after starting Ritalin. Mom brings him to your office on recommendation of the school for escalating behaviors. He recently got into a fight at school and broke up with his girlfriend last night. He is increasingly oppositional at home and slams doors when upset. Mom states that his behavior scares his younger siblings. This morning, for example, he smashed his computer and punched a hole in his bedroom wall during a "rage" episode, seemingly without warning or provocation.

## Key Points

- Irritability and out-of-control behavior are nonspecific symptoms that can be seen in a myriad of conditions and diagnoses.

- Assessing the severity of symptoms and determining risk for harm to self or others is paramount.

- Medical causes should be ruled out before considering psychiatric diagnoses – even in the presence of an identifiable psychosocial stressor.

- It is important to differentiate new or transient symptoms from those related to recurrence of a more chronic illness.

- Relation to psychosocial factors such as divorce, bullying, poor peer relations, or physical abuse should be considered.

- It is helpful to gain corroborative information from the school and any other providers to provide insight about behaviors and functioning in different settings.

- Determine the context of symptom presentation in order to accurately diagnose and treat psychiatric disorders.

## Psychiatric Differential Diagnosis*

**Table 1:** Psychiatric Differential Diagnosis for Irritable or Out-of-Control Behavior

| | |
|---|---|
| Adjustment Disorders | |
| Anxiety Disorders | Acute Stress Disorder<br>Posttraumatic Stress Disorder<br>Generalized Anxiety Disorder<br>Substance-Induced Anxiety Disorder<br>Anxiety Disorder Due to General Medical Condition |
| Attention Deficit Hyperactivity Disorder | |
| Delirium | |
| Disruptive Behavior Disorders | Oppositional Defiant Disorder<br>Conduct Disorder |
| Mood Disorders | Major Depressive Disorder<br>Bipolar Disorder<br>Substance-Induced Mood Disorder |
| Psychotic Disorders | First Break of Psychosis<br>Substance-Induced Psychotic Disorder<br>Psychotic Disorder Due to General Medical Condition<br>Substance Use Disorders |
| Substance Use Disorders | |

\* Please note that this is not an exhaustive list of the differential diagnosis. Diagnoses are limited to those that are most applicable, those that you can assess and treat in a primary care office, or those that should not be overlooked due to risk for harm. See Chapter 1 for additional information.

## Using the Assessment Algorithm

•   In working through this algorithm, please remember that patients can have comorbid conditions. For example, the adolescent who tests positive for opiate use may also be in the midst of a depression and have a history of panic attacks and posttraumatic stress disorder. For this reason, the algorithm does not reach a place that states "STOP." It is recommended that even if you find certain pertinent positives as you go through the algorithm, you should still work your way through it to ensure that other important diagnoses are not overlooked.

•   For the patient presenting with irritable or out-of-control behavior, assessing whether the patient is an imminent danger to self or others is paramount. See Appendix B for a suicide and risk assessment. If the patient is deemed to be an imminent danger, this is an emergent case, and the patient should be referred for psychiatric evaluation at your local emergency room or crisis service.

- If the patient is not an imminent danger, begin your evaluation of the patient by considering possible medical or neurological etiologies for the patient's symptoms. Endocrine, infectious, CNS, cardiac, and metabolic issues can lead to irritable or out-of-control behavior. Consider the possibility of adverse side effects of current medications. For example, stimulants can sometimes increase aggression and hostility. Appropriately workup and treat any possible medical or neurological causes.

- Consider substance use as a potential etiology and order toxicology screening if substance use is suspected. See Chapter 22 for the evaluation of substance use disorders.

- If the patient has had a waxing and waning mental status or sudden onset of symptoms, consider the possibility of a delirium. These are patients who usually present with a more abrupt pattern of symptom onset. See Chapter 14 for the evaluation of delirium.

- Many times, children and adolescents can present with an irritable mood or out-of-control behavior due to a mood disorder. It is important to note that irritability can be seen in either a depressive episode, a manic episode, or a mixed episode. See Chapter 19 for the evaluation of mood disorders.

- Symptoms of irritability or out-of-control behavior can also be caused by the onset of psychotic symptoms. It is important to distinguish whether the psychotic symptoms emerged in the context of mood symptoms or if they are free standing. See Chapter 20 for the evaluation of psychotic disorders.

- Anxiety symptoms can also manifest with irritable or out-of-control behavior. A child with separation anxiety disorder, for example, may become irritable and inconsolable when mom leaves him at day care. See Chapter 11 for the evaluation of anxiety disorders.

- A child with impulsivity and hyperactivity may appear to be out of control. See Chapter 12 for the evaluation of ADHD.

- If there is an identifiable stressor that may be contributing to the patient's current clinical presentation, an adjustment disorder should be considered. See Chapter 10 for the evaluation of adjustment disorders.

- If the out-of-control behavior occurs in the context of oppositionality, difficulty with authority figures, or a basic disregard of the rights of others, see Chapter 15 for the evaluation of disruptive behavior disorders.

- For patients who have continued irritable or out-of-control symptoms, consider referral to a child and adolescent psychiatrist.

## Assessment Algorithm for Irritable or Out-of-Control Behavior

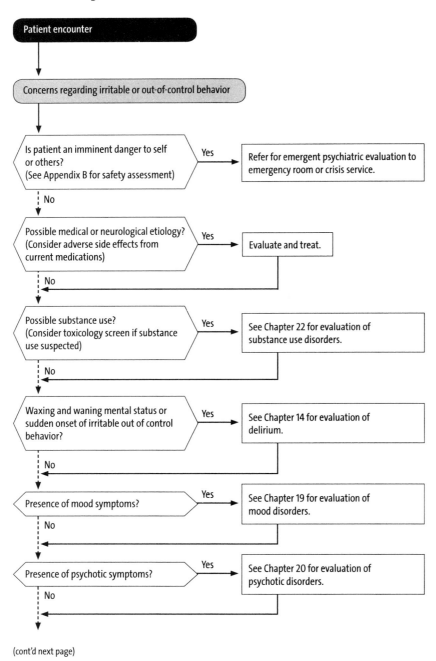

(cont'd next page)

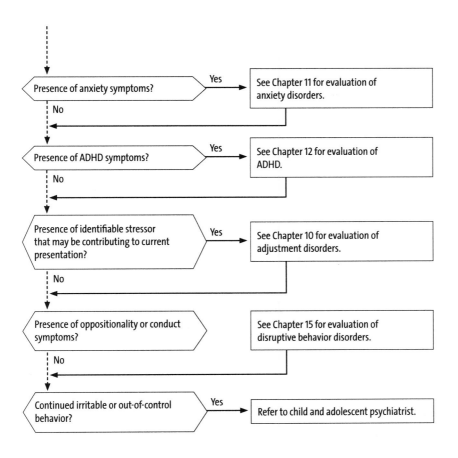

Presence of anxiety symptoms? — Yes → See Chapter 11 for evaluation of anxiety disorders.

No

Presence of ADHD symptoms? — Yes → See Chapter 12 for evaluation of ADHD.

No

Presence of identifiable stressor that may be contributing to current presentation? — Yes → See Chapter 10 for evaluation of adjustment disorders.

No

Presence of oppositionality or conduct symptoms? → See Chapter 15 for evaluation of disruptive behavior disorders.

No

Continued irritable or out-of-control behavior? — Yes → Refer to child and adolescent psychiatrist.

**Take Home Messages**

- Irritability or out-of-control behavior can be quite unnerving for the patient. We have had children tell us about how horrible they feel after the fact, how much they dislike the feeling of losing control, and how they often can't tell when they are about to explode.

- Parents also have a lot of difficulty with irritable or out-of-control behaviors. From the pain and frustration of seeing your child having such a mega-meltdown to feelings of failure as a parent in helping your child regulate behavior, parents often present with a palpable sense of powerlessness, frustration, and desperation. Siblings often report feeling quite scared and not knowing when the next eruption will occur.

- It is important to validate the feelings that the child, parents, and family may be having. Having a primary care provider who understands where they are at can be quite helpful.

- It is important to remain nonjudgmental throughout the work-up and to make sure that the parents do not feel blamed. Having an excellent therapeutic alliance with the child and the family is key to implementing change. Explaining a rationale for working-up this chief complaint can also be helpful.

- If you have seen similar presentations in other patients, it sometimes helps to let them know that. All too often, the child and their parents feel that they are the only ones with this issue.

# 4 Fatigue or Changes in Appetite

## Clinical Snapshots

Billy is a seven-year-old boy with no significant past medical history who is brought in by mom due to concerns about his appetite recently. Mom states that Billy usually eats well and has always been at the 90th percentile for height and weight during past visits to the doctor. She has noticed that for the past two weeks he has become much more picky regarding foods and has even started saying "no" to some of his favorite foods. He has been complaining of feeling tired after school and has started taking afternoon naps again. Mom denies that he has been depressed, but states that he is generally more withdrawn, doesn't play with friends, no longer enjoys playing soccer, and keeps apologizing to mom for being "bad."

Samantha is a 14-year-old girl with no significant past medical history. She is a straight "A" student who enjoys swimming and is on a competitive gymnastics team. She likes to prepare meals for the family and has started pushing mom to "go organic" with her food choices. Mom expresses concern about her tough gymnastics schedule and the pressure to maintain a certain weight. She has noticed Samantha making comments about "feeling fat" and needing to "exercise for four hours to burn off those calories." Mom does not think that she is restricting her food intake or is engaging in any compensatory behaviors to lose weight. Mom is concerned about her daughter as a few of the older girls on the team seem particularly thin.

## Key Points

- Fatigue or changes in appetite are nonspecific symptoms that can be seen in a myriad of conditions and diagnoses. Be sure to clarify the nature, duration, and severity of the symptoms.

- Assessing the severity of symptoms and determining risk for harm to self or others is paramount.

- Medical causes should be ruled out before considering psychiatric diagnoses – even in the presence of an identifiable psychosocial stressor.

- Assess sleep patterns and dietary history (including walking the patient through a day's worth of "normal meals"). Ask about past psychiatric history and family history of psychiatric illness.

- Note the age of the child, the presence of any medical or psychiatric comorbidity, and the functional effects of the symptoms on the child and family.

- It is important to differentiate new or transient symptoms from those related to recurrence of a more chronic illness.

🔑  It is helpful to gain corroborative information from the school and any other providers to provide insight about behaviors and functioning in different settings.

🔑  Determine the context of symptom presentation in order to accurately diagnose and treat psychiatric disorders.

## Psychiatric Differential Diagnosis*

**Table 1:** Psychiatric Differential Diagnosis for Fatigue or Changes in Appetite

| | |
|---|---|
| Adjustment Disorders | |
| Anxiety Disorders | Acute Stress Disorder<br>Posttraumatic Stress Disorder<br>Generalized Anxiety Disorder<br>Substance-Induced Anxiety Disorder<br>Anxiety Disorder Due to General Medical Condition |
| Eating Disorders | Anorexia Nervosa<br>Bulimia Nervosa<br>Eating Disorder NOS |
| Mood Disorders | Major Depressive Disorder<br>Bipolar Disorder<br>Substance-Induced Mood Disorder |
| Psychotic Disorders | First Break of Psychosis<br>Substance-Induced Psychotic Disorder<br>Psychotic Disorder Due to General Medical Condition |
| Somatoform Disorders | |
| Substance Use Disorders | |

\* Please note that this is not an exhaustive list of the differential diagnosis. Diagnoses are limited to those that are most applicable, those that you can assess and treat in a primary care office, or those that should not be overlooked due to risk for harm. See Chapter 1 for additional information.

## Using the Assessment Algorithm

• In working through this algorithm, please remember that patients can have comorbid conditions. For example, the adolescent who is restricting food may also be having panic attacks and fatigue due to worsening of a depressive episode. For this reason, the algorithm does not reach a place that states "STOP". It is recommended that even if you find certain pertinent positives as you go through the algorithm, you should still work your way through it to ensure that other important diagnoses are not overlooked.

- For the patient presenting with fatigue or changes in appetite, assessing whether the patient is an imminent danger to self or others is paramount. Although this chief complaint is not one that immediately strikes you as being at risk for self-harm, consider the case of fatigued patient with no appetite who is suffering from a worsening depression and has developed daily suicidal ideation for the past week. The difficulty in psychiatry is that the patient, for many reasons, may walk in and not list the most clinically concerning symptom as the chief complaint. It is important to develop a structured method for conducting your assessments. See Appendix B for a suicide and risk assessment. If the patient is deemed to be an imminent danger, this is an emergent case, and the patient should be referred for psychiatric evaluation at your local emergency room or crisis service.

- If the patient is not an imminent danger, begin your evaluation of the patient by considering possible medical or neurological etiologies for the patient's symptoms. Consider the possibility of adverse side effects of current medications. For example, stimulants can sometimes cause a decrease in appetite. Appropriately workup and treat any possible medical or neurological causes.

  - The use of many common medications can lead to fatigue or changes in appetite. In particular, hypnotics, muscle relaxants, some anti-depressants, anti-psychotics, and opioids frequently produce sedation as a side effect. Also, those drugs that may interfere with normal sleep patterns, such as stimulants or SSRI anti-depressants, can indirectly lead to fatigue due to decreased sleep. Stimulants may also decrease appetite, while many other psychotropic medications (especially anti-psychotics and anti-depressants) often increase appetite and result in significant weight gain.

- Consider substance use as a potential etiology and order toxicology screening if substance use is suspected. See Chapter 22 for the evaluation of substance use disorders.

- Many times, children and adolescents can present with fatigue or changes in appetite due to a mood disorder. See Chapter 19 for the evaluation of mood disorders.

- Symptoms of fatigue or changes in appetite can also be caused by the onset of psychotic symptoms. It is important to distinguish whether the psychotic symptoms emerged in the context of mood symptoms or if they are free standing. See Chapter 20 for the evaluation of psychotic disorders.

- Eating disorders can present with fatigue or changes in appetite as the chief complaint. This concern may not be voiced by the patient, but rather, may be coming from observations of the parent. See Chapter 16 for the evaluation of eating disorders.

- Anxiety symptoms can also manifest with fatigue or changes in appetite. A child with generalized anxiety disorder, for example, may become so overcome with anxiety that it causes a loss of appetite or fatigue. See Chapter 11 for the evaluation of anxiety disorders.

- Youth with physical complaints, such as fatigue, should be considered for the presence of somatoform disorders. See Chapter 21 for the evaluation of somatoform disorders.

- If there is an identifiable stressor that may be contributing to the patient's current clinical presentation, an adjustment disorder should be considered. See Chapter 10 for the evaluation of adjustment disorders.

- For patients that have continued fatigue or changes in appetite, consider referral to a child and adolescent psychiatrist.

## Assessment Algorithm for Fatigue or Changes in Appetite

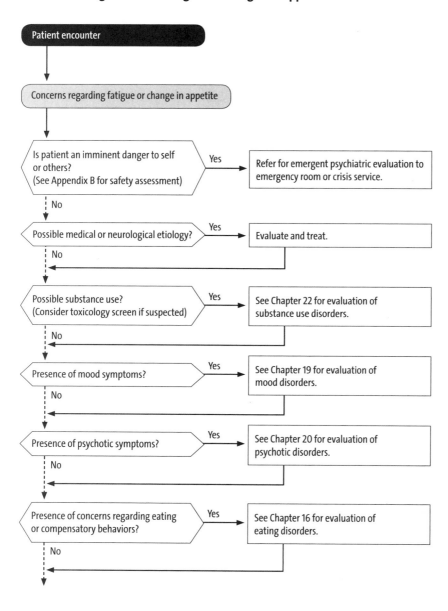

(cont'd next page)

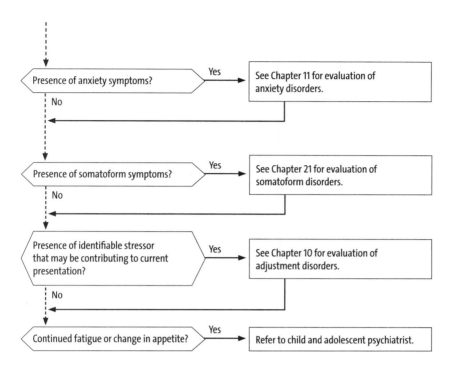

**Take Home Messages**

- Fatigue or changes in appetite are quite nonspecific symptoms that can be related to a wide spectrum of medical and psychiatric illnesses.

- Having a systematic method of working up these chief complaints and conveying the steps ahead can be reassuring for the child as well as the parents. In giving reassurance, ask parents and the child what they are concerned about. Throughout the work-up and treatment of fatigue or changes in appetite, sometimes the most reassuring comment you can make is that the child has had an appropriate medical work-up and that the current symptoms are not due to some undiagnosed life-threatening disease.

- It is important to validate the concerns of the child, parents, and family. Having a primary care provider who understands where they are at can be quite helpful.

- It is important to remain nonjudgmental throughout the work-up and to make sure that the parents do not feel blamed. Having an excellent therapeutic alliance with the child and the family is key to implementing change.

# 5 School Refusal

## Clinical Snapshots

Tyler is a six-year-old boy with no significant past medical history who presents to your office with his mom. She states that it has been getting harder and harder to get him ready for school in the morning, particularly on Mondays. She recalls that he had a tendency to cry when dropped off at daycare, but never quite to this extent. He has begun complaining of a "tummy ache" regularly and has missed nine days of school in the past three weeks. He tends to cling to mom when the school bus arrives and cries regularly.

Amanda is a 15-year-old girl with a history of asthma who is brought in by mom after a concerning phone call from the school guidance counselor. Amanda has not been in school for the past three weeks. She has been cutting classes and is at risk of failing multiple classes. Teachers have noticed that she has been increasingly withdrawn and isolative. She has been seen with a new group of friends and has started smoking pot and drinking beer. She denies any suicidal ideation, but does admit to hopelessness.

## Key Points

- School refusal can be both disruptive and stressful for children, families, teachers, and school administrators. It can have a significant impact on the child's social, emotional, and educational development.

- School refusal is marked by a wide range of behaviors from occasionally bargaining to miss a day of school to completely being absent from school for periods of time. Variations include skipping certain classes, chronic tardiness, and tantrum behaviors. Having a detailed history of the school refusal behaviors is imperative (see Table 1).

- School refusal peaks during the transition to elementary school, middle school, and high school. School refusal can flare-up after weekends, school vacations, or acute stressors such as the death of a pet.

- It is often associated with comorbid psychiatric disorders such as anxiety, depressive, and disruptive behavior disorders.

- Treatment of any underlying or comorbid disorders is necessary to aid in successful remission of school refusal behaviors.

- The work-up and treatment of school refusal is best done in collaboration with the parents and school personnel.

- Prompt response to school refusal is imperative to interrupt its progression. The longer a child stays out of school, the harder it will be to treat school refusal.

**Table 1:** Initial Questions When Evaluating School Refusal

When did your child first start refusing to attend school?
How did it begin?
Have there been any other changes in your child's behavior?
What does your child say about not wanting to go to school?
Has your child ever refused school before?
Is your child disobeying rules at home and/or in school?
Is your child having any trouble at school?
Is your child complaining of any aches or pains?
Does your child seem emotionally upset at the prospect of attending school?
How is your child's mood in general?
How is your child doing academically?
How is your child doing socially?
Have there been any recent changes in the home, school, or other important settings?
How is the family functioning?

## Psychiatric Differential Diagnosis*

**Table 2:** Psychiatric Differential Diagnosis for School Refusal

| Adjustment Disorders | |
|---|---|
| Anxiety Disorders | Acute Stress Disorder |
| | Posttraumatic Stress Disorder |
| | Separation Anxiety Disorder |
| | Panic Disorder |
| | Generalized Anxiety Disorder |
| | Specific Phobia |
| | Social Phobia |
| | Substance-Induced Anxiety Disorder |
| | Anxiety Disorder Due to General Medical Condition |
| Attention Deficit Hyperactivity Disorder | |
| Disruptive Behavior Disorders | Oppositional Defiant Disorder |
| | Conduct Disorder |
| Mood Disorders | Major Depressive Disorder |
| | Bipolar Disorder |
| | Substance-Induced Mood Disorder |
| Substance Use Disorders | |
| Learning Disorders | |
| Mental Retardation | |

* Please note that this is not an exhaustive list of the differential diagnosis. Diagnoses are limited to those that are most applicable, those that you can assess and treat in a primary care office, or those that should not be overlooked due to risk for harm. See Chapter 1 for additional information.

## Using the Assessment Algorithm

- In working through this algorithm, please remember that patients can have comorbid conditions. For example, a first grader being bullied at school may also have a learning disability and separation anxiety. For this reason, the algorithm does not reach a place that states "STOP". It is recommended that even if you find certain pertinent positives as you go through the algorithm, you should still work your way through it to ensure that other important diagnoses are not overlooked.

- For the patient presenting with school refusal, assessing whether the patient is an imminent danger to self or others is paramount. Youths who are being bullied at school, for example, may begin refusing to go to school. The concern about safety arises when that child brings a knife to school for protection or revenge. See Appendix B for a suicide and risk assessment. If the patient is deemed to be an imminent danger, this is an emergent case, and the patient should be referred for psychiatric evaluation at your local emergency room or crisis service.

- If the patient is not an imminent danger, begin your evaluation of the patient by considering possible medical or neurological etiologies for the patient's symptoms. Consider the possibility of adverse side effects of current medications. For example, a child who taking an atypical antipsychotic may refuse to go to school due to over-sedation in the early morning. Appropriately workup and treat any possible medical or neurological causes.

- Consider substance use as a potential etiology and order toxicology screening if substance use is suspected. Patients with substance problems commonly start losing motivation to attend school or decrease their participation in regular activities. See Chapter 22 for the evaluation of substance use disorders.

- Children and adolescents can present with school refusal due to a mood disorder. For example, the child who is depressed starts to isolate and withdraw leading to school refusal. See Chapter 19 for the evaluation of mood disorders.

- School refusal can also be caused by the onset of psychotic symptoms. An adolescent who believes that kids are talking about him in school and have bugged the classroom may refuse to go to school. It is important to distinguish whether the psychotic symptoms emerged in the context of mood symptoms or if they are free standing. See Chapter 20 for the evaluation of psychotic disorders.

- Anxiety symptoms can also manifest with school refusal. A child who has panic disorder with agoraphobia, for example, may be scared to leave the home and may stop attending school. See Chapter 11 for the evaluation of anxiety disorders.

- A child with impulsivity and behavioral problems at school may refuse to attend school as well. See Chapter 12 for the evaluation of ADHD.

- If the school refusal occurs in the context of oppositionality, difficulty with authority figures, or a basic disregard of the rights of others, see Chapter 15 for the evaluation of disruptive behavior disorders.

- If there is an identifiable stressor that may be contributing to the patient's current clinical presentation, an adjustment disorder should be considered. See Chapter 10 for the evaluation of adjustment disorders.

- For patients that have continued school refusal symptoms, consider referral to a child and adolescent psychiatrist.

## Assessment Algorithm for School Refusal*

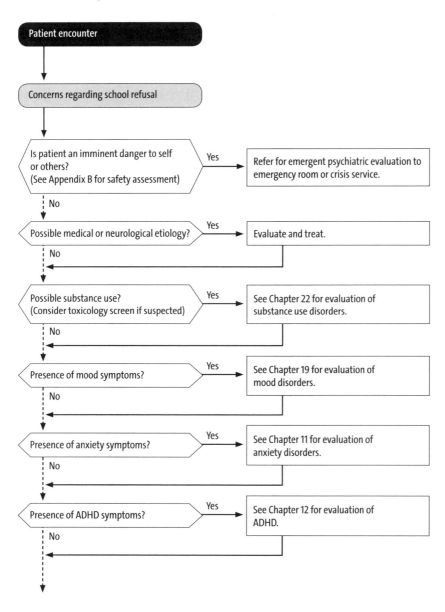

(cont'd next page)

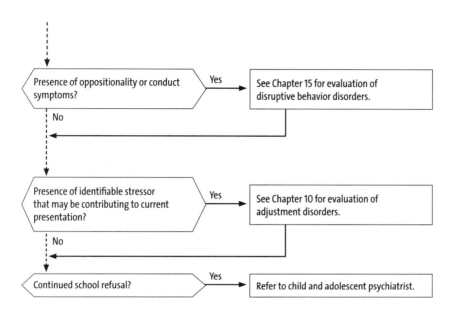

---

\* All patients with school refusal should be considered for the presence of learning disorders (see Chapter 17), mental retardation (see Chapter 18), or other educational difficulties leading to school refusal behavior.

## Treatment Interventions for School Refusal:

- The primary treatment goal for youth with school refusal is early return to school. Physicians should avoid writing excuses for children to stay out of school unless a medical condition makes it necessary for them to stay home.

- As many physical complaints may be associated with school refusal, it is important to rule out medical etiologies. Having the child and the parents understand that you have done a thorough work up will be important in later steps of treatment. You may need to explain that the problem is a manifestation of psychological distress. Often times, communicating this to the school nurse will also be important as headaches and belly aches become common ways to avoid going to the classroom or to get a parent to take them home.

- Treatment should also address comorbid psychiatric problems, family dysfunction and other contributing issues. A multimodal, collaborative team approach should include the physician, the child, parents, school staff, and a mental health professional. Treatment options include education and consultation, behavior strategies, family interventions, and possibly pharmacotherapy for underlying psychiatric disorders. Factors that have been proved effective for treatment improvement are parental involvement and exposure to school. However, few controlled studies have evaluated the efficacy of most treatments.

- A range of empirically supported exposure-based treatment options are available in the management of school refusal. When a child is younger and displays minimal symptoms of fear, anxiety, and depression, working directly with parents and school personnel without direct intervention with the child may suffice in treating the structure and holding environment to keep them in school.

- If the child's difficulties include prolonged school absence, comorbid psychiatric diagnosis, and/or deficits in social skills, active involvement of the child with all other key players is indicated.

- Behavior approaches for the treatment of school refusal are primarily exposure-based. Studies have shown that repeated exposure to feared objects or situations reduces fear and increases exposure attempts in adults. These techniques have been used to treat children with phobias and school refusal. Behavioral techniques focus on a child's behaviors rather than intrapsychic conflict and emphasize treatment in the context of the family and school.

    - These include systematic desensitization (i.e., graded exposure to the school environment), relaxation training, emotive imagery, contingency management, and social skills training.

    - Cognitive behavioral therapy is a highly structured approach that includes specific instructions for children to help gradually increase their exposure to the school environment. In cognitive behavioral therapy, children are encouraged to confront their fears and are taught how to modify negative thoughts.

- Traditional educational and supportive therapy has been shown to be as effective as behavioral therapy for the management of school refusal.

    - Educational-support therapy is a combination of informational presentations and supportive psychotherapy. Children are encouraged to talk about their fears and identify differences between fear, anxiety, and phobias. Children are given information to help them overcome their fears about attending school. They are given written assignments that are discussed at follow-up sessions. Children keep a daily diary to describe their fears, thoughts, coping strategies, and feelings associated with their fears. Unlike cognitive behavioral therapy, children do not receive specific instructions on how to confront their fears, nor do they receive positive reinforcement for school attendance.

- Child therapy involves individual sessions that incorporate relaxation training (to help the child when he or she approaches the school grounds or is questioned by peers), cognitive therapy (to reduce anxiety-provoking thoughts and provide coping statements), social skills training (to improve social competence and interactions with peers), and desensitization (i.e., graded in vivo exposure or emotive imagery).

- Parental involvement and caregiver training are critical factors in enhancing the effectiveness of behavior treatment.

  - Parent-teacher interventions include clinical sessions with parents and consultation with school personnel. Parents are given behavior-management strategies such as escorting the child to school, providing positive reinforcement for school attendance, and decreasing positive reinforcement for staying home (i.e., not watching television while home from school).

  - Parents also benefit from cognitive training to help reduce their own anxiety and understand their role in helping their children make effective changes.

  - School consultation involves specific recommendations to school staff to prepare for the child's return, use of positive reinforcement, and academic, social, and emotional accommodations.

- Pharmacological treatment may be considered for the treatment of underlying psychiatric diagnoses such as a mood disorder or anxiety disorder. Please refer to the corresponding diagnosis and treatment chapters for whichever disorders you are considering. There is no specific medication for the treatment of school refusal.

## Take Home Messages

- School refusal can be difficult for the child as well as the entire family. It is important to provide support to parents so that they can stabilize daily routines for all of their children.

- It is essential to obtain information from teachers and parents in addition to patients. While parents and teachers are more likely to observe the impact of symptoms, only the child can report on the internal distress.

- Children with school refusal can have many physical complaints related to the anxiety of attending school. It is helpful to reassure parents about the health of their child. In some situations, it may be helpful to also point out that prolonged absence from school can negatively impact their child's development, social skills, education, and self-esteem.

- It is important to validate the feelings that the child, parents, and family may be having. Having a primary care provider who understands where they are at can be quite helpful.

- Having an excellent therapeutic alliance with the child and the family is key to implementing change. Explaining a rationale for working-up this chief complaint can also be helpful.

# 6 Recurrent Mild Medical Complaints

## Clinical Snapshots

Vicky is a six-year-old girl who presents to your office about every 2–4 weeks with vague complaints of pain. She does have a history of recurrent ear infections and has had bilateral PE-tube placement. She presents today with "belly pain" for the past week. She is unable to localize her pain, but states that it is worse in the morning. It is a constant dull pain with intermittent sharp pains in the left lower quadrant. During the sharp pains, she has had nausea, but no significant vomiting. She has not had any fever, constipation, or diarrhea. Mom states feeling quite guilty for not taking her complaints more seriously at the beginning as Vicky's abdominal pain seemed particularly worse on school days or when she was asked to do chores. Mom thought that she was "just faking it," but became concerned last night when Vicky was "doubled over" in pain and started "shrieking" in tears.

Billy is a 12-year-old boy with no significant medical history who presents with a chief complaint of recurrent headaches. There is a history of both migraines and seizures in the family. He is otherwise healthy and has had no significant medical illness. Mom states that he has recently been out of it since she and his dad separated three weeks ago. She is concerned that his headaches have increased in intensity and frequency as dad has come over to check up on him and even slept over twice to help comfort him.

## Key Points

- When evaluating a child with recurrent mild medical complaints, the first step is to keep in mind that the suffering of the child and the family is real.

- It is necessary to first rule out an underlying medical condition. Even in the most "obvious" case of somatization, be careful not to overlook a thorough physical exam and judicious work-up.

- Patients with somatic complaints most commonly present with headaches, low energy, pain, sore muscles, abdominal pain, or gastrointestinal symptoms.

- It is important to note whether the patient has a history of multiple somatic complaints, whether there have been multiple physician visits, whether there is a family member with chronic symptoms, whether the child is experiencing psychosocial dysfunction (family, peers, school), as well as, whether these symptoms allow the patient to take on a specific role in the family.

- Note that a psychiatric diagnosis can also coexist with physical illness. If coexisting with physical illness, the impairment is often in excess of what would be expected from the known illness.

Psychiatric diagnoses, such as somatization disorder, are not solely diagnoses of exclusion. Patients need to meet criteria for the psychiatric diagnosis including positive psychiatric symptoms and psychopathology. Having a negative medical workup is not sufficient. For example, 10–40% of patients with conversion disorder were later found to have a physical illness which explained the original symptom.

## Psychiatric Differential Diagnosis*

**Table 1:** Psychiatric Differential Diagnosis for Recurrent Mild Medical Complaints

| | |
|---|---|
| Adjustment Disorders | |
| Anxiety Disorders | Acute Stress Disorder<br>Posttraumatic Stress Disorder<br>Generalized Anxiety Disorder<br>Substance-Induced Anxiety Disorder<br>Anxiety Disorder Due to General Medical Condition |
| Mood Disorders | Major Depressive Disorder<br>Bipolar Disorder<br>Substance-Induced Mood Disorder |
| Psychotic Disorders | First Break of Psychosis<br>Substance-Induced Psychotic Disorder<br>Psychotic Disorder Due to General Medical Condition |
| Somatoform Disorders | Conversion Disorder<br>Somatization Disorder<br>Hypochondriasis<br><br>Also consider factitious disorders and malingering (Note: They are not formally considered somato-form disorders) |
| Substance Use Disorders | |

\* Please note that this is not an exhaustive list of the differential diagnosis. Diagnoses are limited to those that are most applicable, those that you can assess and treat in a primary care office, or those that should not be overlooked due to risk for harm. See Chapter 1 for additional information.

## Using the Assessment Algorithm

- In working through this algorithm, please remember that patients can have comorbid conditions. For example, the school-age child with recurrent abdominal pain may also be in the midst of a depressive episode due to parents' divorce and be experiencing the onset of anxiety symptoms. For this reason, the algorithm does not reach a place that states "STOP". It is recommended that even if you find certain pertinent positives as you go through the algorithm, that you still work your way through it to ensure that other important diagnoses are not overlooked.

- For the patient presenting with recurrent mild medical complaints, assessing whether the patient is an imminent danger to self or others is paramount. Although this chief complaint is not one that immediately strikes you as being at risk for self harm, consider the case of a patient with nonspecific pain symptoms who is suffering from worsening somatic delusions and has developed homicidal ideation towards his teacher for attempting to poison him. The difficulty in psychiatry is that the patient, for many reasons, may walk in and not list the most clinically concerning symptom as the chief complaint. It is important to develop a structured method for conducting your assessments. See Appendix B for a suicide and risk assessment. If the patient is deemed to be an imminent danger, this is an emergent case, and the patient should be referred for psychiatric evaluation at your local emergency room or crisis service.

- If the patient is not an imminent danger, begin your evaluation of the patient by considering possible medical or neurological etiologies for the patient's symptoms. Consider the possibility of adverse side effects of current medications. Appropriately workup and treat any possible medical or neurological causes.

- Consider substance use as a potential etiology and order toxicology screening if substance use is suspected. See Chapter 22 for the evaluation of substance use disorders.

- Many times, children and adolescents can present with recurrent mild medical complaints due to a mood disorder. See Chapter 19 for the evaluation of mood disorders.

- Symptoms, such as pain or bodily dysfunction, can also be caused by the onset of psychotic symptoms. It is important to distinguish whether the psychotic symptoms emerged in the context of mood symptoms or if they are free standing. See Chapter 20 for the evaluation of psychotic disorders.

- Anxiety symptoms can also manifest with recurrent mild medical complaints. A child with generalized anxiety disorder, for example, may become overcome with anxiety causing recurrent nausea and vomiting. See Chapter 11 for the evaluation of anxiety disorders.

- Youths with recurrent mild medical complaints should be considered for the presence of somatoform disorders. Also consider factitious disorders and malingering. See Chapter 21 for the evaluation of somatoform disorders.

- If there is an identifiable stressor that may be contributing to the patient's current clinical presentation, an adjustment disorder should be considered. See Chapter 10 for the evaluation of adjustment disorders.

- For patients that have continued recurrent mild medical complaints, consider referral to a child and adolescent psychiatrist.

## Assessment Algorithm for Recurrent Mild Medical Complaints

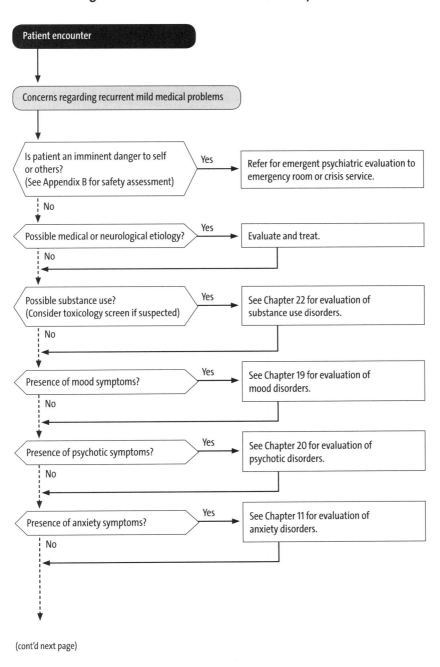

Patient encounter

Concerns regarding recurrent mild medical problems

Is patient an imminent danger to self or others?
(See Appendix B for safety assessment) — Yes → Refer for emergent psychiatric evaluation to emergency room or crisis service.

No

Possible medical or neurological etiology? — Yes → Evaluate and treat.

No

Possible substance use?
(Consider toxicology screen if suspected) — Yes → See Chapter 22 for evaluation of substance use disorders.

No

Presence of mood symptoms? — Yes → See Chapter 19 for evaluation of mood disorders.

No

Presence of psychotic symptoms? — Yes → See Chapter 20 for evaluation of psychotic disorders.

No

Presence of anxiety symptoms? — Yes → See Chapter 11 for evaluation of anxiety disorders.

No

(cont'd next page)

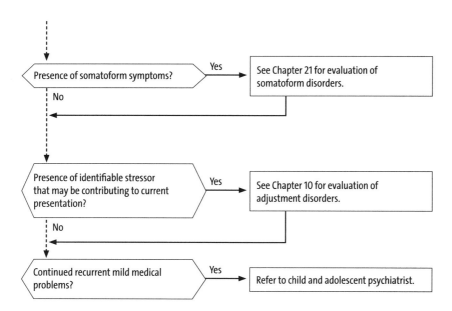

### Take Home Messages

- It is important to build trust with both the patient and the parents. They need to understand that you are taking their concerns seriously and will methodically make sure that medical issues are identified and treated.

- Using examples of mind–body connections like "having butterflies in the stomach" can help patients and parents understand how psychological conflict can manifest with physical symptoms.

- When developing the treatment plan, set clear goals based on functional improvements. Do not base successful treatment on "curing" the ailment.

- Placebo treatments and deception should be avoided. However, during acute episodes, the use of benign, face-saving remedies such as lotions, vitamins, or heating pads could be seen as supportive and facilitative to healing.

- Similarly, making physician contact contingent on being actively sick should be avoided. Scheduled routine appointments with reassurance and positive praise for healthy outcomes should be reinforced.

- Allowing the patient to be an active participant in management of the condition empowers the youths to take ownership of health (as opposed to being afflicted with the mystery debilitating illness).

# 7 Speech Problems or Refusing to Speak

## Clinical Snapshots

Amanda is a six-year-old girl with a history of mild hearing loss due to repeated ear infections. She is brought in by her parents due to concerns about delayed speech and shy, withdrawn behavior at school. Her parents state that she is able to communicate verbally at home. In school, she tends to avoid interactions with the other children; preferring to play near them, but not with them. Attempts by the teacher to reward speaking in class have only been met with more resistance from Amanda. Her family history is significant for panic disorder in mom and generalized anxiety disorder in dad. The parents are concerned about how they can help her to talk in school.

Billy is a three-year-old boy presenting for a well child checkup. Mom denies any current concerns, but states that he isn't particularly affectionate. He tends to keep to himself, plays with the same dinosaur toy for hours, and does not like being hugged. He tends to use a limited vocabulary of words and only mom can understand what he is saying. Upon questioning, mom has a puzzled look as she can not remember a time when he has pointed at objects. She asks you whether this is something to be worried about.

## Key Points

- Concerns about a child's speech often cause parents to bring the child in to the pediatrician's office. The child may present as a toddler who is not yet speaking, a preschooler whose is no longer speaking or seems to have lost language skills, or a school-age child who speaks well in some settings and is silent in others.

- Assessing the severity of symptoms and determining risk for harm to self or others is paramount.

- Medical causes should be ruled out before considering psychiatric diagnoses – even in the presence of an identifiable psychosocial stressor.

- It is helpful to gain corroborative information from the school and any other providers to provide insight about behaviors and functioning in different settings.

- Determine the context of symptom presentation in order to accurately diagnose and treat psychiatric disorders.

## Psychiatric Differential Diagnosis*

**Table 1:** Psychiatric Differential Diagnosis for Speech Problems or Refusal to Speak

| | | |
|---|---|---|
| Adjustment Disorders | | |
| Autism and Pervasive Developmental Disorders | Autistic Disorder<br>Asperger's Disorder<br>Childhood Disintegrative Disorder<br>Rett's Disorder | |
| Anxiety Disorders | Acute Stress Disorder<br>Posttraumatic Stress Disorder<br>Generalized Anxiety Disorder<br>Obsessive Compulsive Disorder<br>Selective Mutism<br>Substance-Induced Anxiety Disorder<br>Anxiety Disorder Due to General Medical Condition | |
| Delirium | | |
| Disruptive Behavior Disorders | Oppositional Defiant Disorder<br>Conduct Disorder | |
| Learning Disorders | | |
| Mental Retardation | | |
| Mood Disorders | Major Depressive Disorder<br>Bipolar Disorder<br>Substance-Induced Mood Disorder | |
| Psychotic Disorders | First Break of Psychosis<br>Substance-Induced Psychotic Disorder<br>Psychotic Disorder Due to General Medical Condition | |
| Substance Use Disorders | | |

* Please note that this is not an exhaustive list of the differential diagnosis. Diagnoses are limited to those that are most applicable, those that you can assess and treat in a primary care office, or those that should not be overlooked due to risk for harm. See Chapter 1 for additional information.

## Using the Assessment Algorithm

- In working through this algorithm, please remember that patients can have comorbid conditions. For example, the child who tests positive for hearing loss may also have autism. For this reason, the algorithm does not reach a place that states "STOP." It is recommended that even if you find certain pertinent positives as you go through the algorithm, you should still work your way through it to ensure that other important diagnoses are not overlooked.

- For the patient presenting with speech problems or refusing to speak, assessing whether the patient is an imminent danger to self or others is paramount. See Appendix B for a suicide and risk assessment. If the patient is deemed to be an imminent danger, this is an emergent case, and the patient should be referred for psychiatric evaluation at your local emergency room or crisis service.

- If the patient is not an imminent danger, begin your evaluation of the patient by considering possible medical or neurological etiologies for the patient's symptoms. For the toddler who has never spoken, hearing, communication development, global development, and physical abnormalities need to be assessed. Consider the possibility of adverse side effects of current medications. Appropriately workup and treat any possible medical or neurological causes.

- Consider substance use as a potential etiology and order toxicology screening if substance use is suspected. See Chapter 22 for the evaluation of substance use disorders.

- If the patient has had a waxing and waning mental status or sudden onset of symptoms, consider the possibility of a delirium. These are patients who usually present with a more abrupt pattern of symptom onset. See Chapter 14 for the evaluation of delirium.

- Many times, children and adolescents can present with speech problems or refusal to speak due to a mood disorder. Major depression in children usually presents with irritability, sleep disturbance, decreased enjoyment of activities, and some social withdrawal. Occasionally, a child will develop a more classically adult-style melancholic depression, which may include speaking little or not at all. Such a silence can be distinguished from the other etiologies previously discussed by the accompanying affective abnormalities and the ability to talk sufficiently when prompted. See Chapter 19 for the evaluation of mood disorders.

- Symptoms of speech problems or refusal to speak can also be caused by the onset of psychotic symptoms. It is important to distinguish whether the psychotic symptoms emerged in the context of mood symptoms or if they are free standing. See Chapter 20 for the evaluation of psychotic disorders.

- Anxiety symptoms can also manifest with speech problems or refusal to speak. An acutely traumatized child may stop speaking for a period of time immediately after the trauma. A suddenly silent child who appears affectively numbed, fearful, or hyperaroused, should be gently questioned with and without parents in the room for recent traumatic experiences. See Chapter 11 for the evaluation of anxiety disorders.

- Global developmental delay is the most common cause of delayed onset of speech, as a child with a low IQ will take longer to develop language skills. See Chapter 18 for evaluation of mental retardation, as well as Chapter 17 for the evaluation of learning disorders.

- A child who has had a normal appearing development and now presents with loss of verbal and social skills, especially reciprocal social interest, joint attention, and imaginative play, requires assessment for autism and pervasive developmental disorders (see Chapter 13).

    - Assessment using a standardized tool may be helpful. A Checklist for Autism in Toddlers (CHAT) is for children less than 24 months, while the M-CHAT is for children 24–36 months old.

    - The Social Communication Questionnaire, a 10-minute parent-completed questionnaire, can be used to screen for pervasive developmental disorders in children of 4 years and older.

- If there is an identifiable stressor that may be contributing to the patient's current clinical presentation, an adjustment disorder should be considered. See Chapter 10 for the evaluation of adjustment disorders.

- If the speech problems or refusal to speak occurs in the context of oppositionality, difficulty with authority figures, or a basic disregard of the rights of others, see Chapter 15 for the evaluation of disruptive behavior disorders.

- For patients that have continued speech problems or refusal to speak, consider referral to a child and adolescent psychiatrist.

## Assessment Algorithm for Speech Problems or Refusing to Speak*

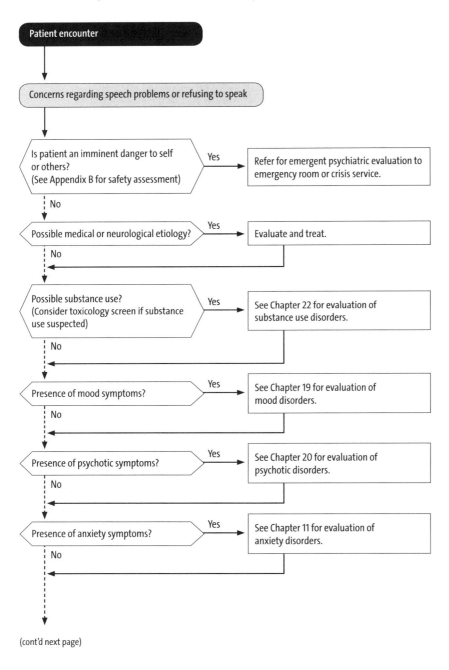

(cont'd next page)

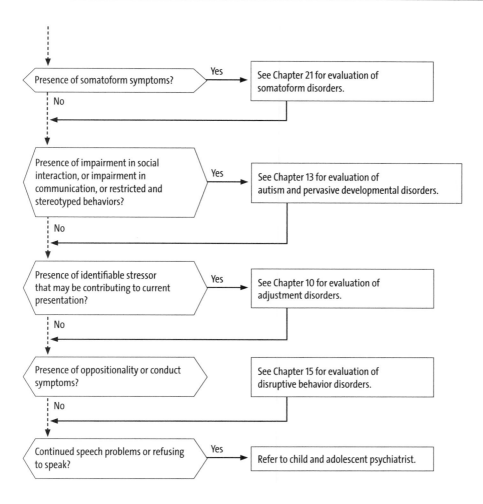

---

* Patients with speech problems or refusal to speak should be considered for the presence of motor, receptive, or cognitive issues which may impact ability to speak or ability to learn how to speak. Also see Chapter 17 for evaluation of learning disorders and Chapter 18 for evaluation of mental retardation.

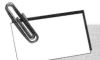

### Take Home Messages

- Speech problems or refusal to speak can be caused by a wide spectrum of medical and psychiatric illnesses.

- Having a systematic method of working up these chief complaints and conveying the steps ahead can be reassuring for the child as well as the parents.

- It is important to validate the concerns of the child, parents, and family. Having a primary care provider who understands where they are at can be helpful.

- As a child's speech development and ability to communicate are essential to appropriate development, prompt evaluation and treatment are necessary to prevent the child from developing other developmental problems.

# 8 Sudden Personality Change or Confusion

## Clinical Snapshots

John is a 17-year-old boy with a history of asthma who presents due to a sudden change in behavior. His father brings him in and states that John just took his final exams yesterday. Everything seemed fine, until he went out with a few of his high school friends to celebrate. When he returned home, dad noticed that he stumbled through the door and was making some bizarre statements. John denies any alcohol or drug use and says that he was at a party where other kids were "being stupid." He continues to plead that he has not used any substances.

Tara is a 12-year-old girl with no significant past medical history whom you diagnosed with a urinary tract infection two days ago. Mom calls you frantically stating that she has developed a fever of 102 degrees Fahrenheit, has been acting strange and appears confused. Mom denies any side effects from the antibiotic you had prescribed and states that Tara has been taking it regularly. Mom became more concerned when Tara started speaking to her with unintelligible nonsense words and started talking about the scary man standing outside her second floor bedroom window. Mom states that Tara also has interspersed moments of being "normal" again and seems to snap out of it just as quickly as this began.

## Key Points

- Any acute change in personality or signs of confusion, particularly in the presence of disorientation or a fluctuating level of consciousness, should be evaluated emergently.

- Assessing the severity of symptoms and determining risk for harm to self or others is paramount. It is important to factor risk for unintended harm during episodes of confusion.

- Medical causes should be ruled out before considering psychiatric diagnoses – even in the presence of an identifiable psychosocial stressor.

## Psychiatric Differential Diagnosis*

**Table 1:** Psychiatric Differential Diagnosis for Sudden Personality Change or Confusion

| | |
|---|---|
| Adjustment Disorders | |
| Anxiety Disorders | Acute Stress Disorder<br>Posttraumatic Stress Disorder<br>Generalized Anxiety Disorder<br>Substance-Induced Anxiety Disorder<br>Anxiety Disorder Due to General Medical Condition |
| Mood Disorders | Major Depressive Disorder<br>Bipolar Disorder<br>Substance-Induced Mood Disorder |
| Psychotic Disorders | First Break of Psychosis<br>Substance-Induced Psychotic Disorder<br>Psychotic Disorder Due to General Medical Condition |
| Substance Use Disorders | |

\* Please note that this is not an exhaustive list of the differential diagnosis. Diagnoses are limited to those that are most applicable, those that you can assess and treat in a primary care office, or those that should not be overlooked due to risk for harm. See Chapter 1 for additional information.

## Using the Assessment Algorithm

- In working through this algorithm, please remember that patients can have comorbid conditions. For example, the adolescent who tests positive for opiate use and is in the midst of a worsening depression may now be presenting with delirium due to carbon monoxide poisoning after a failed suicide attempt. For this reason, the algorithm does not reach a place that states "STOP." It is recommended that even if you find certain pertinent positives as you go through the algorithm, that you still work your way through it to ensure that other important diagnoses are not overlooked.

- For the patient presenting with sudden personality change or confusion, assessing whether the patient is an imminent danger to self or others is paramount. Although the patient may not necessarily voice suicidality or homicidality, the potential for impulsive or dangerous behavior during any episode of confusion must be considered. It is important to develop a structured method for conducting your assessments. See Appendix B for a suicide and risk assessment. If the patient is deemed to be an imminent danger, this is an emergent case, and the patient should be referred for psychiatric evaluation at your local emergency room or crisis service.

- If the patient is not an imminent danger, begin your evaluation of the patient by considering possible medical or neurological etiologies for the patient's symptoms. Sudden personality change or confusion should be initially worked up to rule out any potentially life-threatening medical causes. Consider the possibility of adverse side effects of current medications. Appropriately workup and treat any possible medical or neurological causes.

- Consider substance use as a potential etiology and order toxicology screening if substance use is suspected. See Chapter 22 for the evaluation of substance use disorders.

- Delirium is characterized by a fluctuating course, disorientation, impaired memory, decreased attention, altered sleep wake cycle, perceptual disturbances, motor abnormalities, EEG changes, and disorganized thoughts, behaviors, and speech. See Chapter 14 for a discussion of delirium.

- Youths with mood disorders can present with personality changes. See Chapter 19 for the evaluation of mood disorders.

- Symptoms, such as personality change or confusion, can also be caused by the onset of psychotic symptoms. It is important to distinguish whether the psychotic symptoms emerged in the context of mood symptoms or if they are free standing. See Chapter 20 for the evaluation of psychotic disorders.

- Anxiety symptoms can also manifest with personality changes or confusion. A child with obsessive compulsive disorder, for example, may become preoccupied with mental rituals and appear confused. See Chapter 11 for the evaluation of anxiety disorders.

- If there is an identifiable stressor that may be contributing to the patient's current clinical presentation, an adjustment disorder should be considered. See Chapter 10 for the evaluation of adjustment disorders.

- For patients that have continued personality change or confusion, consider referral to a child and adolescent psychiatrist.

## Assessment Algorithm for Sudden Personality Change or Confusion

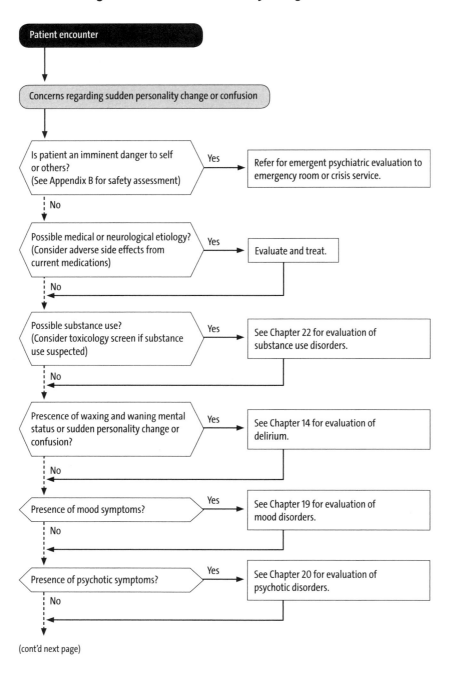

(cont'd next page)

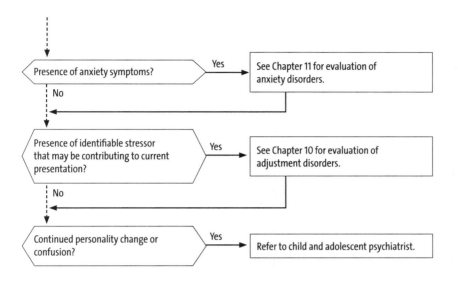

# 9 Excessive Worries

## Clinical Snapshots

Ethan is a four-year-old boy with a history of failure to thrive and was adopted from a Russian orphanage two years ago. He has made substantial gains nutritionally, but continues to be at the 25th percentile for height and weight. Mom presents to your office expressing concern about his shy, timid nature and his frequent worrying. She explains that he has nightmares about twice a week and will become "much clingier" the following morning. This is usually followed by temper tantrums the following morning when he is dropped off for daycare. The daycare staff report that he spends the first couple of hours preoccupied about multiple ways that mom may get into an accident and is soon in tears, having convinced himself that she will not return.

Olivia is a 13-year-old girl with a history of cystic fibrosis. She has had multiple medical hospitalizations and was recently discharged four days ago after a two week stay due to shortness of breath. She is brought in by dad for a follow-up visit. During this appointment, she mentions to you that she has been feeling more sad lately. She has been thinking about her family, her dad's recent layoff, how her mom worries too much about her, and how she will keep up with her schoolwork. She states that she has been worrying about things like this "for years," but has recently been having "anxiety attacks." She goes on to explain that when she worries about these things too much, she starts feeling overwhelmed. "All of a sudden" she notes, she will start feeling short of breath, her heart starts pounding, and her hands become sweaty. She starts thinking that something bad will happen and is fearful that she will stop breathing.

## Key Points

- Excessive worries can occur with a number of different psychiatric diagnoses. A patient with worries does not always have an anxiety disorder.

- Although anxiety disorders are one of the most common diagnoses in children and adolescents, it is important to rule out other etiologies of the symptoms before jumping to a specific diagnosis. It is important to keep in mind a broad differential diagnosis when examining and talking with these children and their families. For example, it is important not to miss the child with excessive worries due to a worsening mood disorder.

- Alternatively, not all children with anxiety disorders will present with a chief complaint of worrying.

- Youths with worries can present in a variety of ways. For example, they can present with physical symptoms, such as headache or belly pain, or school refusal, nightmares, or decreased social or academic functioning.

It is beneficial to gather as much information from the patient, parents, and teachers which will help you not only in diagnosis but in determining the severity of the situation.

## Psychiatric Differential Diagnosis*

**Table 1:** Psychiatric Differential Diagnosis for Excessive Worries

| | |
|---|---|
| Adjustment Disorders | |
| Anxiety Disorders | Acute Stress Disorder<br>Posttraumatic Stress Disorder<br>Generalized Anxiety Disorder<br>Substance-Induced Anxiety Disorder<br>Anxiety Disorder Due to General Medical Condition<br>Selective Mutism<br>Panic Disorder |
| Mood Disorders | Major Depressive Disorder<br>Bipolar Disorder<br>Substance-Induced Mood Disorder |
| Psychotic Disorders | First Break of Psychosis<br>Substance-Induced Psychotic Disorder<br>Psychotic Disorder Due to General Medical Condition |
| Somatoform Disorders | Conversion Disorder<br>Somatization Disorder<br>Hypochondriasis<br><br>Also consider factitious disorders and malingering (Note: They are not formally considered somato-form disorders) |
| Substance Use Disorders | |

\* Please note that this is not an exhaustive list of the differential diagnosis. Diagnoses are limited to those that are most applicable, those that you can assess and treat in a primary care office, or those that should not be overlooked due to risk for harm. See Chapter 1 for additional information.

## Using the Assessment Algorithm

- In working through this algorithm, please remember that patients can have comorbid conditions. For example, the child who has posttraumatic stress disorder can also be in the midst of a depression and have a history of panic attacks. For this reason, the algorithm does not reach a place that states "STOP." It is recommended that even if you find certain pertinent positives as you go through the algorithm, that you still work your way through it to ensure that other important diagnoses are not overlooked.

- For the patient presenting with excessive worries, assessing whether the patient is an imminent danger to self or others is paramount. Although this chief complaint is not one that immediately strikes you as being at risk for self harm, consider the case of patient with multiple worries who is suffering from worsening persecutory delusions who is planning to kill himself as he sees no other way out. The difficulty in psychiatry is that the patient, for many reasons, may walk in and not list the most clinically concerning symptom as the chief complaint. It is important to develop a structured method for conducting your assessments. See Appendix B for a suicide and risk assessment. If the patient is deemed to be an imminent danger, this is an emergent case, and the patient should be referred for psychiatric evaluation at your local emergency room or crisis service.

- If the patient is not an imminent danger, begin your evaluation of the patient by considering possible medical or neurological etiologies for the patient's symptoms. Consider the possibility of adverse side effects of current medications. Certain medications, such as stimulants or antidepressants, can increase anxiety symptoms. Appropriately workup and treat any possible medical or neurological causes.

- Consider substance use as a potential etiology and order toxicology screening if substance use is suspected. See Chapter 22 for the evaluation of substance use disorders.

- Many times, children and adolescents can present with excessive worries due to a mood disorder. See Chapter 19 for the evaluation of mood disorders.

- Symptoms, such as worries or anxiety, can also be caused by the onset of psychotic symptoms. It is important to distinguish whether the psychotic symptoms emerged in the context of mood symptoms or if they are free standing. See Chapter 20 for the evaluation of psychotic disorders.

- Anxiety disorders can also manifest with excessive worries. As noted above, although anxiety disorders are one of the most common diagnoses in youths, it is important to rule out other etiologies of the symptoms before jumping to an anxiety disorder diagnosis. Youths may also present with more than one specific anxiety disorder. See Chapter 11 for the evaluation of anxiety disorders.

- Children and adolescents with excessive worries should be considered for the presence of somatoform disorders. They may present with excessive worries, but their worries could deal with excessive bodily concerns. Also consider factitious disorders and malingering. See Chapter 21 for the evaluation of somatoform disorders.

- If there is an identifiable stressor that may be contributing to the patient's current clinical presentation, an adjustment disorder should be considered. See Chapter 10 for the evaluation of adjustment disorders. It is important not to underestimate how much a child's anxiety may stem from an undiagnosed learning disorder or other academic difficulty.

- For patients that have continued excessive worries, consider referral to a child and adolescent psychiatrist.

## Assessment Algorithm for Excessive Worries

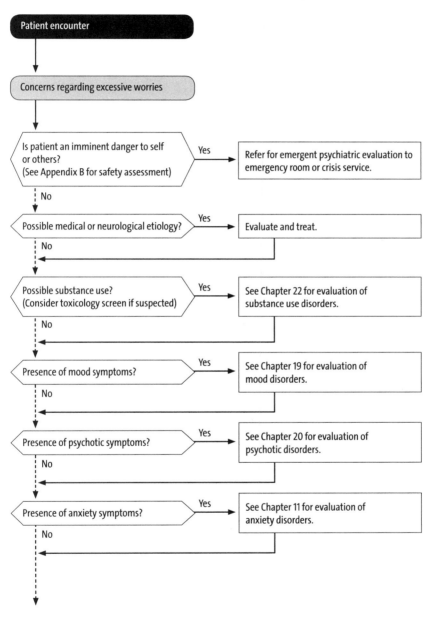

Patient encounter

Concerns regarding excessive worries

Is patient an imminent danger to self or others?
(See Appendix B for safety assessment) — Yes → Refer for emergent psychiatric evaluation to emergency room or crisis service.

No

Possible medical or neurological etiology? — Yes → Evaluate and treat.

No

Possible substance use?
(Consider toxicology screen if suspected) — Yes → See Chapter 22 for evaluation of substance use disorders.

No

Presence of mood symptoms? — Yes → See Chapter 19 for evaluation of mood disorders.

No

Presence of psychotic symptoms? — Yes → See Chapter 20 for evaluation of psychotic disorders.

No

Presence of anxiety symptoms? — Yes → See Chapter 11 for evaluation of anxiety disorders.

No

(cont'd next page)

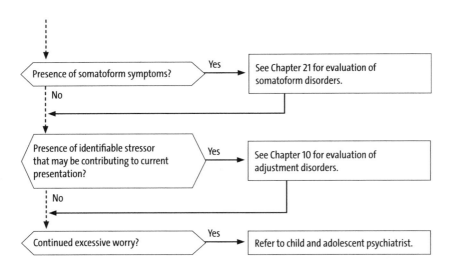

# Section III
# Psychiatric Diagnoses

This section presents information related to accurately diagnosing psychiatric illnesses and determining severity of symptoms. Each chapter provides an *assessment algorithm* based upon DSM-IV-TR and a *severity assessment and treatment algorithm* to determine the level of intervention required. Your clinical input will help lead you through the algorithm to the relevant portions of the book regarding the treatment options in subsequent sections. As you become more familiar with these diagnoses, you may find yourself referring only to the algorithm or going directly to the treatment section.

This section reviews the following diagnoses:

- Adjustment Disorders
- Anxiety Disorders
- Attention Deficit Hyperactivity Disorder
- Autism and Pervasive Development Disorders
- Delirium
- Disruptive Behavior Disorders
- Eating Disorders
- Learning Disorders
- Mental Retardation
- Mood Disorders
- Psychotic Disorders
- Somatoform and Factitious Disorders
- Substance Use Disorders

# 10 Adjustment Disorder

**Diagnosis Discussed in this Chapter:**

- Adjustment Disorder

Adjustment disorder is diagnosed when the patient is exhibiting symptoms or behaviors that are related to the onset of a specific identifiable stressor. The prevalence of adjustment disorder in youth ranges between 2% and 8%.

Adjustment Disorder is defined by the DSM-IV-TR as the development of emotional or behavioral symptoms within three months of experiencing a stressful event. These symptoms may cause either distress out of proportion from what would be expected from the stressor, or cause a significant impairment in social or academic functioning. Common stressors for children include a change in home life such as divorce, birth of a sibling, a change in schools, or physical illness. In adolescents, relationship issues such as the breakup with a girlfriend or boyfriend is a common stressor. Importantly, these symptoms do not represent bereavement. Adjustment disorders are transient and symptoms do not persist beyond six months after the removal of the stressor.

Children and adolescents with an adjustment disorder may present with depressed mood, anxiety, or disturbance of conduct. Comorbidity with depression and anxiety is common, therefore it is important to screen for and treat these conditions as necessary. Please refer to the appropriate diagnostic and treatment chapters for further information.

Treatment with brief supportive psychotherapy may be useful for a child with an adjustment disorder. In addition, cognitive behavioral therapy may help improve coping skills and future response to stress. Psychotherapeutic interventions are discussed in Chapter 29. Psychosocial interventions to alleviate environmental stressors or provide additional supports to the patient and family can be particularly helpful. They are discussed further in Chapter 30.

## Assessment Algorithm

As only one diagnosis is discussed in this chapter, a diagnostic algorithm is not presented. Diagnostic criteria are reviewed below.

## Diagnostic Criteria

### Adjustment Disorder

A.  The development of emotional or behavioral symptoms in response to an identifiable stressor(s) occurring within 3 months of the onset of the stressor(s).

B.  These symptoms or behaviors are clinically significant as evidenced by either of the following:
    (1)   marked distress that is in excess of what would be expected from exposure to the stressor
    (2)   significant impairment in social or occupational (academic) functioning

C.  The stress-related disturbance does not meet the criteria for another specific Axis I disorder and is not merely an exacerbation of a preexisting Axis I or Axis II disorder.

D.  The symptoms do not represent Bereavement.

E.  Once the stressor (or its consequences) has terminated, the symptoms do not persist for more than an additional 6 months.

*Specify* if:
    **Acute:**   if the disturbance lasts less than 6 months
    **Chronic:**   if the disturbance lasts for 6 months or longer

Adjustment Disorders are coded based on the subtype, which is selected according to the predominant symptoms. The specific stressor(s) can be specified on Axis IV.

| | |
|---|---|
| **309.0** | **With Depressed Mood** |
| **309.24** | **With Anxiety** |
| **309.28** | **With Mixed Anxiety and Depressed Mood** |
| **309.3** | **With Disturbance of Conduct** |
| **309.4** | **With Mixed Disturbance of Emotions and Conduct** |
| **309.9** | **Unspecified** |

Reprinted with the permission from the Diagnostic and Statistical Manual of Mental Disorders, Fourth Edition, Text Revison (© 2000), American Psychiatric Association.

## Severity Assessment and Treatment Algorithm

Please refer to Figure 1 for the severity assessment and treatment algorithm for adjustment disorders.

**Figure 1:** Severity Assessment and Treatment Algorithm for Adjustment Disorders

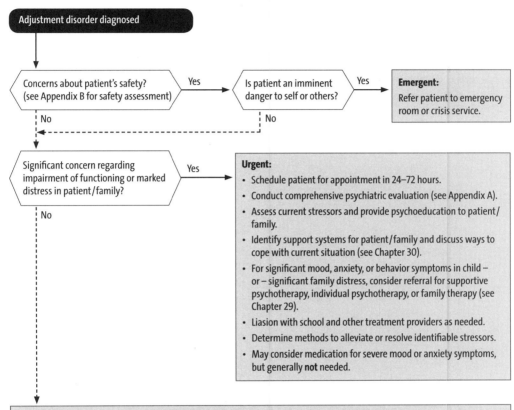

– See appropriate chapters for assessment of anxiety or mood symptoms
– See treatments in Section IV for additional information regarding interventions

## Grief and Bereavement

The death of a family member and other significant losses can illicit a severe behavioral response in children. In addition, a bereaved child may often experience irritability along with depressed mood, social withdrawal, a decline in academic performance, and sleep disturbance. If symptoms are present two months after the loss or severity significantly elevates (for example, the child becomes suicidal), an assessment for Major Depressive Disorder or another Axis I diagnosis should be considered. Routine treatment includes support of the child and the family. Often times, a conversation regarding how people deal with loss can be helpful. Likewise, normalizing the experience and letting people know what to expect is also well received. Close monitoring for more severe symptoms of anxiety or depression should occur on a continuing basis until the stressor has resolved and the symptoms have subsided. Emergent treatment is necessary if there is a significant impairment in functioning or if symptoms of psychosis or suicidality occur.

# 11 Anxiety Disorders

**Diagnoses Discussed in this Chapter:**

- Acute Stress Disorder
- Posttraumatic Stress Disorder
- Separation Anxiety Disorder
- Generalized Anxiety Disorder
- Social Phobia
- Specific Phobia
- Panic Disorder with or without Agoraphobia
- Obsessive Compulsive Disorder
- Anxiety Disorder Not Otherwise Specified (NOS)

---

- Selective Mutism
    - Classified in DSM-IV as a "Disorder First Diagnosed in Infancy, Childhood, or Adolescence"

Anxiety disorders are among the most common psychiatric disorders affecting children and adolescents and often go undiagnosed. Epidemiological data indicate that as many as 13% of youth between the ages of 9 and 17 are affected. Nearly 43% of patients with a chief complaint of school refusal are found to have a comorbid anxiety disorder.

The proper evaluation of a child or adolescent should begin by obtaining a thorough history from both the parent and child in order to assess the quality, onset, duration, and degree of impairment from symptoms. A self-report questionnaire (see Appendix E) may be helpful in the assessment and monitoring of symptoms. A clinical interview in which the child and parent are asked about DSM-IV-TR criteria symptoms is invaluable. It provides the opportunity to ask follow-up questions and to gain a more thorough understanding of the patient.

Anxiety disorders in children not only present with a change in behavior or academic performance, but also with somatic complaints such as headaches or abdominal symptoms. Physical conditions that mimic an anxiety disorder must be ruled out. Some examples include hyperthyroidism, high caffeine intake, migraines, seizure disorders, lead poisoning, hypoglycemia, pheochromocytoma, and cardiac arrhythmias.

The abuse of amphetamines, cocaine, hallucinogens, and stimulants can illicit anxiety and irritability in children. Cessation of alcohol, barbiturates, benzodiazepines, and opiates may also cause similar symptoms. Medications may also cause side effects that mimic an anxiety disorder. These can include antiasthmatics, antihistamines, sympathomimetics, steroids, SSRIs, antipsychotics, diet pills, and over the counter cold medications.

If an anxiety disorder is diagnosed, a multimodal treatment approach is recommended. This includes teaching the patient and child about anxiety, consulting the patient's teacher, and considering cognitive-behavioral interventions, psychodynamic psychotherapy, family therapy, and pharmacotherapy. Regarding severity, clinical guidelines suggest that mild anxiety disorder should be treated with psychotherapy initially. The addition of medication is recommended when there is a need for acute symptom reduction, there has only been partial response to psychotherapy, there is a comorbid disorder that requires treatment, or there is the potential for improved outcome with combined treatment. Selective serotonin reuptake inhibitor (SSRI) antidepressants are currently the medication of choice for the treatment of childhood anxiety disorders. Alpha adrenergic agonists and benzodiazepines may also be considered.

Psychotherapy recommendations include cognitive behavioral therapy, psychodynamic psychotherapy, and parent-child or family therapy. For certain disorders, progressive relaxation training and guided imagery have also been effective. Treating parents and families can be essential to clinical improvement of the child since parental anxiety, parenting styles, insecure attachment, and parent-child interactions play an important role in the development and maintenance of childhood anxiety.

Emergent interventions are warranted when suicidal ideation or self-injurious behavior accompanies anxiety symptoms. When safety becomes an imminent concern, emergent psychiatric evaluation should be obtained by referring a patient to the emergency room or crisis service.

## Assessment Algorithm

The assessment algorithm for anxiety disorders is presented in Figure 1. Diagnostic criteria are reviewed below.

**Figure 1:** Assessment Algorithm for Anxiety Disorders

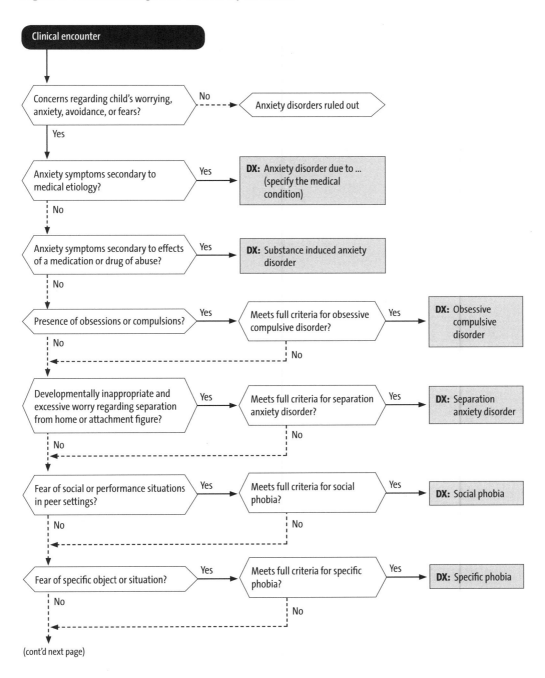

(cont'd next page)

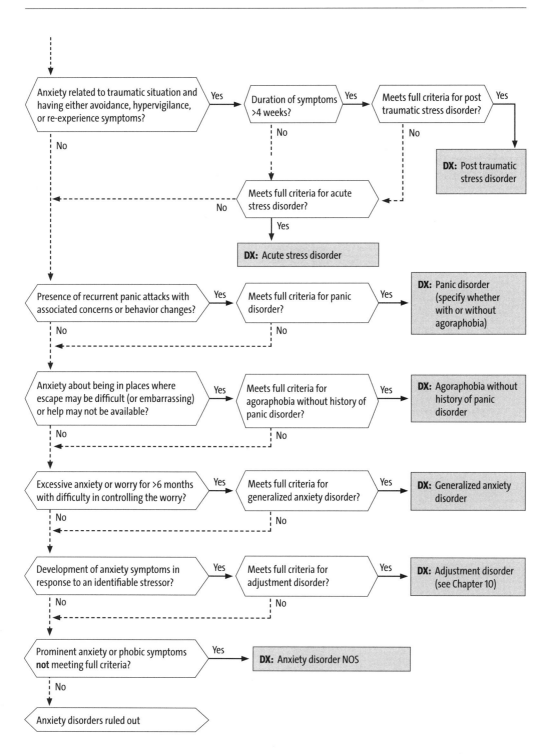

## Diagnostic Criteria

### Acute Stress Disorder

A.  The person has been exposed to a traumatic event in which both of the following were present:

    (1)   the person experienced, witnessed, or was confronted with an event or events that involved actual or threatened death or serious injury, or a threat to the physical integrity of self or others

    (2)   the person's response involved intense fear, helplessness, or horror

B.  Either while experiencing or after experiencing the distressing event, the individual has three (or more) of the following dissociative symptoms:

    (1)   a subjective sense of numbing, detachment, or absence of emotional responsiveness

    (2)   a reduction in awareness of his or her surroundings (e.g., "being in a daze")

    (3)   derealization

    (4)   depersonalization

    (5)   dissociative amnesia (i.e., inability to recall an important aspect of the trauma)

C.  The traumatic event is persistently reexperienced in at least one of the following ways: recurrent images, thoughts, dreams, illusions, flashback episodes, or a sense of reliving the experience; or distress on exposure to reminders of the traumatic event.

D.  Marked avoidance of stimuli that arouse recollections of the trauma (e.g., thoughts, feelings, conversations, activities, places, people).

E.  Marked symptoms of anxiety or increased arousal (e.g., difficulty sleeping, irritability, poor concentration, hypervigilance, exaggerated startle response, motor restlessness).

F.  The disturbance causes clinically significant distress or impairment in social, occupational, or other important areas of functioning or impairs the individual's ability to pursue some necessary task, such as obtaining necessary assistance or mobilizing personal resources by telling family members about the traumatic experience.

G.  The disturbance lasts for a minimum of 2 days and a maximum of 4 weeks and occurs within 4 weeks of the traumatic event.

H.  The disturbance is not due to the direct physiological effects of a substance (e.g., a drug of abuse, a medication) or a general medical condition, is not better accounted for by Brief Psychotic Disorder, and is not merely an exacerbation of a preexisting Axis I or Axis II disorder.

### Posttraumatic Stress Disorder

A.  The person has been exposed to a traumatic event in which both of the following were present:

    (1)   the person experienced, witnessed, or was confronted with an event or events that involved actual or threatened death or serious injury, or a threat to the physical integrity of self or others

    (2)   the person's response involved intense fear, helplessness, or horror. **Note:** In children, this may be expressed instead by disorganized or agitated behavior

B.  The traumatic event is persistently reexperienced in one (or more) of the following ways:

    (1)   recurrent and intrusive distressing recollections of the event, including images, thoughts, or perceptions. **Note:** In young children, repetitive play may occur in which themes or aspects of the trauma are expressed.

    (2)   recurrent distressing dreams of the event. **Note:** In children, there may be frightening dreams without recognizable content.

    (3)   acting or feeling as if the traumatic event were recurring (includes a sense of reliving the experience, illusions, hallucinations, and dissociative flashback episodes, including those that occur on awakening or when intoxicated). **Note:** In young children, trauma-specific reenactment may occur.

    (4)   intense psychological distress at exposure to internal or external cues that symbolize or resemble an aspect of the traumatic event

    (5)   physiological reactivity on exposure to internal or external cues that symbolize or resemble an aspect of the traumatic event

C.  Persistent avoidance of stimuli associated with the trauma and numbing of general responsiveness (not present before the trauma), as indicated by three (or more) of the following:

    (1)   efforts to avoid thoughts, feelings, or conversations associated with the trauma
    (2)   efforts to avoid activities, places, or people that arouse recollections of the trauma
    (3)   inability to recall an important aspect of the trauma
    (4)   markedly diminished interest or participation in significant activities
    (5)   feeling of detachment or estrangement from others
    (6)   restricted range of affect (e.g., unable to have loving feelings)
    (7)   sense of a foreshortened future (e.g., does not expect to have a career, marriage, children, or a normal life span)

D.  Persistent symptoms of increased arousal (not present before the trauma), as indicated by two (or more) of the following:

    (1)   difficulty falling or staying asleep
    (2)   irritability or outbursts of anger
    (3)   difficulty concentrating
    (4)   hypervigilance
    (5)   exaggerated startle response

E.  Duration of the disturbance (symptoms in Criteria B, C, and D) is more than 1 month.

F.  The disturbance causes clinically significant distress or impairment in social, occupational, or other important areas of functioning.

*Specify* if:
    **Acute:**   if duration of symptoms is less than 3 months
    **Chronic:**   if duration of symptoms is 3 months or more

*Specify* if:
    **With Delayed Onset:**   if onset of symptoms is at least 6 months after the stressor

## Separation Anxiety Disorder

A.  Developmentally inappropriate and excessive anxiety concerning separation from home or from those to whom the individual is attached, as evidenced by three (or more) of the following:

    (1)   recurrent excessive distress when separation from home or major attachment figures occurs or is anticipated
    (2)   persistent and excessive worry about losing, or about possible harm befalling, major attachment figures
    (3)   persistent and excessive worry that an untoward event will lead to separation from a major attachment figure (e.g., getting lost or being kidnapped)
    (4)   persistent reluctance or refusal to go to school or elsewhere because of fear of separation
    (5)   persistently and excessively fearful or reluctant to be alone or without major attachment figures at home or without significant adults in other settings
    (6)   persistent reluctance or refusal to go to sleep without being near a major attachment figure or to sleep away from home
    (7)   repeated nightmares involving the theme of separation
    (8)   repeated complaints of physical symptoms (such as headaches, stomachaches, nausea, or vomiting) when separation from major attachment figures occurs or is anticipated

B.  The duration of the disturbance is at least 4 weeks.

C.  The onset is before age 18 years.

D.  The disturbance causes clinically significant distress or impairment in social, academic (occupational), or other important areas of functioning.

E.  The disturbance does not occur exclusively during the course of a Pervasive Developmental Disorder, Schizophrenia, or other Psychotic Disorder and, in adolescents and adults, is not better accounted for by Panic Disorder With Agoraphobia.

*Specify* if:
**Early Onset:**  if onset occurs before age 6 years

## Generalized Anxiety Disorder

A.  Excessive anxiety and worry (apprehensive expectation), occurring more days than not for at least 6 months, about a number of events or activities (such as work or school performance).

B.  The person finds it difficult to control the worry.

C.  The anxiety and worry are associated with three (or more) of the following six symptoms (with at least some symptoms present for more days than not for the past 6 months). **Note:** Only one item is required in children.

    (1)  restlessness or feeling keyed up or on edge
    (2)  being easily fatigued
    (3)  difficulty concentrating or mind going blank
    (4)  irritability
    (5)  muscle tension
    (6)  sleep disturbance (difficulty falling or staying asleep, or restless unsatisfying sleep)

D.  The focus of the anxiety and worry is not confined to features of an Axis I disorder, e.g., the anxiety or worry is not about having a Panic Attack (as in Panic Disorder), being embarrassed in public (as in Social Phobia), being contaminated (as in Obsessive-Compulsive Disorder), being away from home or close relatives (as in Separation Anxiety Disorder), gaining weight (as in Anorexia Nervosa), having multiple physical complaints (as in Somatization Disorder), or having a serious illness (as in Hypochondriasis), and the anxiety and worry do not occur exclusively during Posttraumatic Stress Disorder.

E.  The anxiety, worry, or physical symptoms cause clinically significant distress or impairment in social, occupational, or other important areas of functioning.

F.  The disturbance is not due to the direct physiological effects of a substance (e.g/a drug of abuse, a medication) or a general medical condition (e.g., hyperthyroidism) and does not occur exclusively during a Mood Disorder, a Psychotic Disorder, or a Pervasive Developmental Disorder.

## Social Phobia

A.  A marked and persistent fear of one or more social or performance situations in which the persons exposed to unfamiliar people or to possible scrutiny by others. The individual fears that he or she will act in a way (or show anxiety symptoms) that will be humiliating or embarrassing. **Note:** In children, there must be evidence of the capacity for age-appropriate social relationships with familiar people and the anxiety must occur in peer settings, not just in interactions with adults.

B.  Exposure to the feared social situation almost invariably provokes anxiety, which may take the form of a situationally bound or situationally predisposed Panic Attack. **Note:** In children, the anxiety may be expressed by crying, tantrums, freezing, or shrinking from social situations with unfamiliar people.

C.  The person recognizes that the fear is excessive or unreasonable. **Note:** In children, this feature may be absent.

D.  The feared social or performance situations are avoided or else are endured with intense anxiety or distress.

E.  The avoidance, anxious anticipation, or distress in the feared social or performance situation(s) interferes significantly with the person's normal routine, occupational (academic) functioning, or social activities or relationships, or there is marked distress about having the phobia.

F.  In individuals under age 18 years, the duration is at least 6 months.

G.  The fear or avoidance is not due to the direct physiological effects of a substance (e.g., a drug of abuse, a medication) or a general medical condition and is not better accounted for by another mental disorder (e.g., Panic Disorder With or Without Agoraphobia, Separation Anxiety Disorder, Body Dysmorphic Disorder, a Pervasive Developmental Disorder, or Schizoid Personality Disorder).

H.  If a general medical condition or another mental disorder is present, the fear in Criterion A is unrelated to it, e.g., the fear is not of Stuttering, trembling in Parkinson's disease, or exhibiting abnormal eating behavior in Anorexia Nervosa or Bulimia Nervosa.

*Specify* if:
   **Generalized:** if the fears include most social situations (also consider the additional diagnosis of Avoidant Personality Disorder)

## Specific Phobia

A.  Marked and persistent fear that is excessive or unreasonable, cued by the presence or anticipation of a specific object or situation (e.g., flying, heights, animals, receiving an injection, seeing blood).

B.  Exposure to the phobic stimulus almost invariably provokes an immediate anxiety response, which may take the form of a situationally bound or situationally predisposed Panic Attack. **Note:** In children, the anxiety may be expressed by crying, tantrums, freezing, or clinging.

C.  The person recognizes that the fear is excessive or unreasonable. **Note:** In children, this feature may be absent.

D.  The phobic situation(s) is avoided or else is endured with intense anxiety or distress.

E.  The avoidance, anxious anticipation, or distress in the feared situation(s) interferes significantly with the person's normal routine, occupational (or academic) functioning, or social activities or relationships, or there is marked distress about having the phobia.

F.  In individuals under age 18 years, the duration is at least 6 months.

G.  The anxiety, Panic Attacks, or phobic avoidance associated with the specific object or situation are not better accounted for by another mental disorder, such as Obsessive-Compulsive Disorder (e.g., fear of dirt in someone with an obsession about contamination), Posttraumatic Stress Disorder (e.g., avoidance of stimuli associated with a severe stressor), Separation Anxiety Disorder (e.g., avoidance of school), Social Phobia (e.g., avoidance of social situations because of fear of embarrassment), Panic Disorder With Agoraphobia, or Agoraphobia Without History of Panic Disorder.

*Specify* type:
   **Animal Type**
   **Natural Environment Type** (e.g., heights, storms, water)
   **Blood-Injection-Injury Type**
   **Situational Type** (e.g., airplanes, elevators, enclosed places)
   **Other Type** (e.g., fear of choking, vomiting, or contracting an illness; in children, fear of loud sounds or costumed characters)

## Agoraphobia

•  If a person develops anxiety or avoidance related to open spaces or any place outside of the home they can be diagnosed with this anxiety disorder.

## Panic Disorder With Agoraphobia

A.  Both (1) and (2):

   (1)  recurrent unexpected Panic Attacks

   (2)  at least one of the attacks has been followed by 1 month (or more) of one (or more) of the following:

      (a)  persistent concern about having additional attacks

      (b)  worry about the implications of the attack or its consequences (e.g., losing control, having a heart attack, "going crazy")

      (c)  a significant change in behavior related to the attacks

B.  The presence of Agoraphobia.

C.  The Panic Attacks are not due to the direct physiological effects of a substance (e.g., a drug of abuse, a medication) or a general medical condition (e.g., hyperthyroidism).

D.  The Panic Attacks are not better accounted for by another mental disorder, such as Social Phobia (e.g., occurring on exposure to feared social situations), Specific Phobia (e.g., on exposure to a specific phobic situation), Obsessive-Compulsive Disorder (e.g., on exposure to dirt in someone with an obsession about contamination), Posttraumatic Stress Disorder (e.g., in response to stimuli associated with a severe stressor), or Separation Anxiety Disorder (e.g., in response to being away from home or close relatives).

## Panic Disorder without Agoraphobia

•  Criteria met for a Panic Disorder (see above)

•  Patient does not have agoraphobia

## Obsessive-Compulsive Disorder

A.  Either obsessions or compulsions:

*Obsessions as defined by (1), (2), (3), and (4):*

   (1)  recurrent and persistent thoughts, impulses, or images that are experienced, at some time during the disturbance, as intrusive and inappropriate and that cause marked anxiety or distress

   (2)  the thoughts, impulses, or images are not simply excessive worries about reallife problems

   (3)  the person attempts to ignore or suppress such thoughts, impulses, or images, or to neutralize them with some other thought or action

   (4)  the person recognizes that the obsessional thoughts, impulses, or images are a product of his or her own mind (not imposed from without as in thought insertion)

*Compulsions as defined by (1) and (2):*

   (1)  repetitive behaviors (e.g., hand washing, ordering, checking) or mental acts (e.g., praying, counting, repeating words silently) that the person feels driven to perform in response to an obsession, or according to rules that must be applied rigidly

   (2)  the behaviors or mental acts are aimed at preventing or reducing distress or preventing some dreaded event or situation; however, these behaviors or mental acts either are not connected in a realistic way with what they are designed to neutralize or prevent or are clearly excessive

B.  At some point during the course of the disorder, the person has recognized that the obsessions or compulsions are excessive or unreasonable. **Note:** This does not apply to children.

C.  The obsessions or compulsions cause marked distress, are time consuming (take more than 1 hour a day), or significantly interfere with the person's normal routine, occupational (or academic) functioning, or usual social activities or relationships.

D.  If another Axis I disorder is present, the content of the obsessions or compulsions is not restricted to it (e.g., preoccupation with food in the presence of an Eating Disorder; hair pulling in the presence of Trichotillomania; concern with appearance in the presence of Body Dysmorphic Disorder; preoccupation with drugs in the presence of a Substance Use Disorder; preoccupation with having a serious illness in the presence of Hypochondriasis; preoccupation with sexual urges or fantasies in the presence of a Paraphilia; or guilty ruminations in the presence of Major Depressive Disorder).

E.   The disturbance is not due to the direct physiological effects of a substance (e.g., a drug of abuse, a medication) or a general medical condition.

*Specify* if:
   **With Poor Insight:**   if, for most of the time during the current episode, the person does not recognize that the obsessions and compulsions are excessive or unreasonable

### Anxiety Disorder Not Otherwise Specified (NOS)

•   Disorders with prominent anxiety or phobia symptoms not meeting full criteria

The diagnostic criteria for Acute Stress Disorder, Posttraumatic Stress Disorder, Separation Anxiety Disorder, Generalized Anxiety Disorder, Social Phobia, Specific Phobia, Panic Disorder With Agoraphobia, and Obsessive-Compulsive Disorder reprinted with permission from the Diagnostic and Statistical Manual of Mental Disorders, Fourth Edition, Text Revison (© 2000), American Psychiatric Association.

## Severity Assessment and Treatment Algorithm

Please refer to Figure 2 for the severity assessment and treatment algorithm for Anxiety Disorders.

**Figure 2:** Severity Assessment and Treatment Algorithm for Anxiety Disorders

**Anxiety disorder diagnosed**

Concerns about patient's safety? (see Appendix B for safety assessment) — **Yes** → Is patient an imminent danger to self or others? — **Yes** → **Emergent:** Refer patient to emergency room or crisis service.

**No** / **No**

Significant concern regarding impairment of functioning or marked distress in patient/family? — **Yes** →

**Urgent:**
- Schedule patient for appointment in 24–72 hours.
- Conduct comprehensive psychiatric evaluation (see Appendix A).
- Provide psychoeducation to patient/family about diagnosis, what to expect, coping with current difficulties, and treatment plan.
- Refer for cognitive behavior therapy (CBT) (see Chapter 29). If unavailable, refer for individual psychotherapy. Certain anxiety disorders have other evidence based therapies – consult with specialist.
- For moderate to severe anxiety symptoms, start treatment with SSRI medication (see Chapter 24).
- For concern regarding severe anxiety symptoms while awaiting efficacy of SSRI trial, consider use of benzodiazepine (see Chapter 26) or adrenergic agonists (see Chapter 23).
- Liasion with school and other treatment providers as needed.
- Anxiety symptoms may also be present in the parent/siblings, be aware of their needs and identify support systems or treatment providers for them as needed.

**No**

**Routine:**
- Schedule patient for appointment in 3–7 days.
- Conduct comprehensive psychiatric evaluation (see Appendix A).
- Provide psychoeducation to patient/family about diagnosis, what to expect, coping with current difficulties, and treatment plan.
- Refer for cognitive behavior therapy (CBT) (see Chapter 29). If unavailable, refer for individual psychotherapy. Certain anxiety disorders have other evidence based therapies – consult with specialist.
- Consider SSRI trial for moderate to severe anxiety symptoms, if symptoms have not responded to trial of psychotherapy, or for worsening of symptoms (see Chapter 24).
- May consider use of benzodiazepine (see Chapter 26) or adrenergic agonists (see Chapter 23) while awaiting efficacy of SSRI trial, however, generally not needed.
- Liasion with school and other treatment providers as needed.
- Anxiety symptoms may also be present in the parent/siblings, be aware of their needs and identify support systems or treatment providers for them as needed.

– Incorporate routine use of rating scales to monitor treatment progess

## Selective Mutism

Selective Mutism, based upon DSM-IV-TR is not classified as an anxiety disorder. Rather, it is listed as a "Disorder First Diagnosed in Infancy, Childhood, or Adolescence". It is presented in this chapter for its anxiety-related manifestations. Due to its lack of fitting into the overall structure of this text as such, a description of the disorder is presented here in its entirety.

---

### Diagnostic Criteria for Selective Mutism (adapted from the DSM-IV-TR)

- Failing to speak in situations where speech is expected despite speaking in other settings
- Lasting greater than 1 month
- Without concurrent speech pathology

---

Selective mutism usually develops in the context of a child with an inhibited, fearful temperament who displays anxiety and undergoes an environmental stress, such as starting school. The inhibited style is present before onset of mutism. Children with selective mutism often nod, shake their head, grunt, whisper, gesture, or respond with one word answers. The family history is often positive for anxiety disorders, mutism, or extreme shyness in a parent or older sibling. The home is usually where the most consistent speech is heard. Parents may have accommodated to their child's lack of verbal communication to an extraordinary degree, allowing the child to avoid feared situations, be home schooled, or even use sign language.

The evaluation will be primarily done through the parents, as the child is unlikely to speak to the pediatrician or PCP. A premorbid history should be obtained with screening for temperamental style, shorter periods of mutism before onset of the full disorder, current stressors (such as a move to a new home or change in schools), and a familial history of mutism and anxiety.

Particular attention should be paid to whether the child is communicating. A lack of any form of communication, or a lack of joint attention, suggest a more pervasive developmental disorder. Likewise, there is a high rate of comorbidity among anxiety disorders in children, and screening for OCD, PTSD, social phobia, panic disorder, and generalized anxiety disorder should be considered.

Treatments for selective mutism include psychotherapy, pharmacotherapy, behavioral modification, and speech therapy:

- Psychotherapy for selective mutism has historically focused on psychodynamic modalities with the assumption that the mutism was an expression of a trauma or primary relationship disturbance. More recently, with the view that it is an anxiety disorder, psychotherapy has been employed utilizing cognitive behavioral therapy principles.
- Pharmacotherapy may also be considered, with SSRI antidepressant being preferred.
- Behavioral modification and speech therapy for patients without speech pathology have not been shown to be effective treatment modalities, but may be attempted in the face of refractory cases or a lack of other resources.

Additional recommendations include not forcing the child to speak, keeping the child in a regular classroom unless other special needs arise, facilitating peer relationships with small group activities, and providing positive reinforcement for attempts to speak in stressful situations.

- Contact with the school can facilitate many of these goals and prevent erroneous actions, such as removing the child from a regular classroom or placing pressure on the child to speak in class.

# 12 Attention Deficit Hyperactivity Disorder

**Diagnosis Discussed in this Chapter:**

- Attention Deficit Hyperactivity Disorder

Inattention, impulsivity, out of control behavior, and hyperactivity are all common childhood complaints. An evaluation for Attention Deficit Hyperactivity Disorder (ADHD) should be initiated when a child presents with these symptoms along with academic underachievement or behavior problems. It is a diagnosis made by clinical interview. Helpful standardized parent and teacher rating scales are available (see Appendix E for suggested rating scales).

Importantly, the symptoms must be present before the age 7 for a diagnosis of ADHD to be made. Impairment must also be present in two or more settings such as home, school, or daycare. Comorbidity is also common including: Oppositional Defiant Disorder, Conduct Disorder, Learning Disorders, Anxiety Disorder, Mood Disorders, and Substance Abuse.

Routine treatment for mild ADHD includes parent education, behavioral modification, and school consultation. Parents need to provide consistent routines and structure while reducing excessive stimulation. School-related interventions include a 504 plan or individualized educational plan to ensure the child will receive needed services and attention. Classroom and testing modifications can be helpful for those with mild to moderate symptoms. A small and self-contained classroom or resource room with a high teacher to student ratio can be helpful for children with moderate to severe symptoms. Seating the child in front of the room away from distractions, dividing assignments into small segments, and keeping an assignment book may also be helpful. The move from elementary to middle school can be challenging for a child with ADHD and may exacerbate academic and behavior problems, and, therefore, support with academic transitions should be provided (see Chapter 30).

Stimulant medications are FDA approved for use with ADHD (see Chapter 28). Other medications such as atomoxetine (see Chapter 28), alpha adrenergic agents (see Chapter 23), and bupropion (see Chapter 24) may also be considered. Psychotherapeutic interventions can also be considered (see Chapter 29).

Emergent interventions are warranted when suicidal ideation or self-injurious behavior accompanies ADHD symptoms. When safety becomes an imminent concern, emergent psychiatric evaluation should be obtained by referring the patient to the emergency room or crisis service.

## Assessment Algorithm

As only one diagnosis is discussed in this chapter, a diagnostic algorithm is not presented. Diagnostic criteria are reviewed below.

# Diagnostic Criteria

## Attention-Deficit/Hyperactivity Disorder

A.  Either (1) or (2):
  (1)  six (or more) of the following symptoms of inattention have persisted for at least 6 months to a degree that is maladaptive and inconsistent with developmental level:
  *Inattention*
  (a)  often fails to give close attention to details or makes careless mistakes in schoolwork, work, or other activities
  (b)  often has difficulty sustaining attention in tasks or play activities
  (c)  often does not seem to listen when spoken to directly
  (d)  often does not follow through on instructions and fails to finish school-work, chores, or duties in the workplace (not due to oppositional behavior or failure to understand instructions)
  (e)  often has difficulty organizing tasks and activities
  (f)  often avoids, dislikes, or is reluctant to engage in tasks that require sustained mental effort (such as schoolwork or homework)
  (g)  often loses things necessary for tasks or activities (e.g., toys, school assignments, pencils, books, or tools)
  (h)  is often easily distracted by extraneous stimuli
  (i)  is often forgetful in daily activities
  (2)  six (or more) of the following symptoms of **hyperactivity-impulsivity** have persisted for at least 6 months to a degree that is maladaptive and inconsistent with developmental level:
  *Hyperactivity*
  (a)  often fidgets with hands or feet or squirms in seat
  (b)  often leaves seat in classroom or in other situations in which remaining seated is expected
  (c)  often runs about or climbs excessively in situations in which it is inappropriate (in adolescents or adults, may be limited to subjective feelings of restlessness)
  (d)  often has difficulty playing or engaging in leisure activities quietly
  (e)  is often "on the go" or often acts as if "driven by a motor"
  (f)  often talks excessively
  *Impulsivity*
  (g)  often blurts out answers before questions have been completed
  (h)  often has difficulty awaiting turn
  (i)  often interrupts or intrudes on others (e.g., butts into conversations or games)
B.  Some hyperactive-impulsive or inattentive symptoms that caused impairment were present before age 7 years.
C.  Some impairment from the symptoms is present in two or more settings (e.g., at school [or work] and at home).
D.  There must be clear evidence of clinically significant impairment in social, academic, or occupational functioning.
E.  The symptoms do not occur exclusively during the course of a Pervasive Developmental Disorder, Schizophrenia, or other Psychotic Disorder and are not better accounted for by another mental disorder (e.g., Mood Disorder, Anxiety Disorder, Dissociative Disorder, or a Personality Disorder).

*Code* based on type:
  **314.01  Attention-Deficit/Hyperactivity Disorder, Combined Type:** if both Criteria A1 and A2 are met for the past 6 months
  **314.00  Attention-Deficit/Hyperactivity Disorder, Predominantly Inattentive Type:** if Criterion A1 is met but Criterion A2 is not met for the past 6 months
  **314.01  Attention-Deficit/Hyperactivity Disorder, Predominantly Hyperactive-Impulsive Type:** if Criterion A2 is met but Criterion A1 is not met for the past 6 months
**Coding note:**  For individuals (especially adolescents and adults) who currently have symptoms that no longer meet full criteria, "In Partial Remission" should be specified.

## Severity Assessment and Treatment Algorithm

**Figure 1:** Severity Assessment and Treatment Algorithm for ADHD

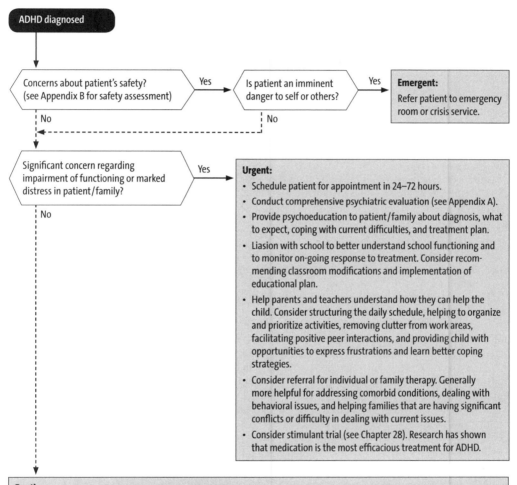

**ADHD diagnosed**

Concerns about patient's safety? (see Appendix B for safety assessment) — Yes → Is patient an imminent danger to self or others? — Yes → **Emergent:** Refer patient to emergency room or crisis service.

No / No

Significant concern regarding impairment of functioning or marked distress in patient/family? — Yes →

**Urgent:**
- Schedule patient for appointment in 24–72 hours.
- Conduct comprehensive psychiatric evaluation (see Appendix A).
- Provide psychoeducation to patient/family about diagnosis, what to expect, coping with current difficulties, and treatment plan.
- Liasion with school to better understand school functioning and to monitor on-going response to treatment. Consider recommending classroom modifications and implementation of educational plan.
- Help parents and teachers understand how they can help the child. Consider structuring the daily schedule, helping to organize and prioritize activities, removing clutter from work areas, facilitating positive peer interactions, and providing child with opportunities to express frustrations and learn better coping strategies.
- Consider referral for individual or family therapy. Generally more helpful for addressing comorbid conditions, dealing with behavioral issues, and helping families that are having significant conflicts or difficulty in dealing with current issues.
- Consider stimulant trial (see Chapter 28). Research has shown that medication is the most efficacious treatment for ADHD.

No

**Routine:**
- Schedule patient for appointment in 3–7 days.
- Plan for intervention is similiar to that for urgent severity.
- Stimulant trial (see Chapter 28) should be considered as research has shown that medication is the most efficacious treatment for ADHD.

– Incorporate routine use of rating scales to monitor treatment progess

# 13 Autism and Pervasive Developmental Disorders

## Diagnoses Discussed in this Chapter:

- Autistic Disorder
- Asperger's Disorder
- Childhood Disintegrative Disorder
- Rett's Disorder
- Pervasive Developmental Disorder Not Otherwise Specified (NOS)

Pervasive developmental disorders are diagnosed when the patient is exhibiting severe impairment that is pervasive in both social and psychological development. In children with autistic disorder, there is a substantial delay in communication and social interaction. In addition, there is the development of restricted, repetitive, or stereotypic behavior, interests, and activities.

Asperger's Disorder differs in that children with this disorder have normal language and cognitive development. There is a significant delay in social interaction and the development of restricted interests and repetitive behaviors and activities.

In comparison, children with Childhood Disintegrative Disorder have seemingly normal development for the first two years of life. Children then lose skills in language, play, and bowel control. Their social interactions become impaired and they develop restrictive, repetitive, stereotyped behaviors.

Lastly, with Rett's Disorder, children are born with normal head circumference and have seemingly normal development for the first five months after birth. They then lose previously acquired skills and can become severely impaired.

The assessment and treatment of autism and pervasive developmental disorders requires a multidisciplinary team. Early identification of children at risk is paramount as early intervention may lead to improved outcomes. Advocating for comprehensive services and managing comorbid psychiatric disorders can be invaluable.

## Assessment Algorithm

The assessment algorithm for autism and pervasive developmental disorders is presented in Figure 1. Diagnostic criteria are reviewed below and are adapted from the DSM-IV-TR.

**Figure 1:** Assessment Algorithm for Autism and Pervasive Developmental Disorders

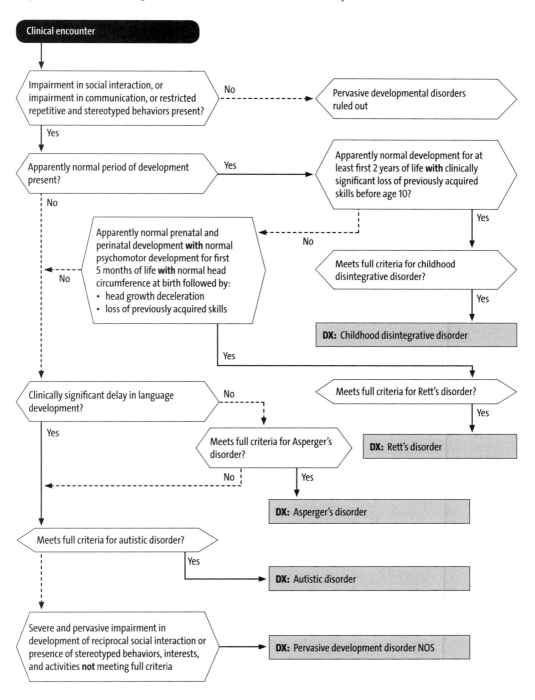

## Diagnostic Criteria

### Autistic Disorder

A.  A total of six (or more) items from (1), (2), and (3), with at least two from (1), and one each from (2) and (3):
    (1)  qualitative impairment in social interaction, as manifested by at least two of the following:
         (a)  marked impairment in the use of multiple nonverbal behaviors such as eye-to-eye gaze, facial expression, body postures, and gestures to regulate social interaction
         (b)  failure to develop peer relationships appropriate to developmental level
         (c)  a lack of spontaneous seeking to share enjoyment, interests, or achievements with other people (e.g., by a lack of showing, bringing, or pointing out objects of interest)
         (d)  lack of social or emotional reciprocity
    (2)  qualitative impairments in communication as manifested by at least one of the following:
         (a)  delay in, or total lack of, the development of spoken language (not accompanied by an attempt to compensate through alternative modes of communication such as gesture or mime)
         (b)  in individuals with adequate speech, marked impairment in the ability to initiate or sustain a conversation with others
         (c)  stereotyped and repetitive use of language or idiosyncratic language
         (d)  lack of varied, spontaneous make-believe play or social imitative play appropriate to developmental level
    (3)  restricted repetitive and stereotyped patterns of behavior, interests, and activities, as manifested by at least one of the following:
         (a)  encompassing preoccupation with one or more stereotyped and restricted patterns of interest that is abnormal either in intensity or focus
         (b)  apparently inflexible adherence to specific, nonfunctional routines or rituals
         (c)  stereotyped and repetitive motor mannerisms (e.g., hand or finger flapping or twisting, or complex whole-body movements)
         (d)  persistent preoccupation with parts of objects
B.  Delays or abnormal functioning in at least one of the following areas, with onset prior to age 3 years: (1) social interaction, (2) language as used in social communication, or (3) symbolic or imaginative play.
C.  The disturbance is not better accounted for by Rett's Disorder or Childhood Disintegrative Disorder.

### Asperger's Disorder

A.  Qualitative impairment in social interaction, as manifested by at least two of the following:
    (1)  marked impairment in the use of multiple nonverbal behaviors such as eye-to-eye gaze, facial expression, body postures, and gestures to regulate social interaction
    (2)  failure to develop peer relationships appropriate to developmental level
    (3)  a lack of spontaneous seeking to share enjoyment, interests, or achievements with other people (e.g., by a lack of showing, bringing, or pointing out objects of interest to other people)
    (4)  lack of social or emotional reciprocity
B.  Restricted repetitive and stereotyped patterns of behavior, interests, and activities, as manifested by at least one of the following:
    (1)  encompassing preoccupation with one or more stereotyped and restricted patterns of interest that is abnormal either in intensity or focus
    (2)  apparently inflexible adherence to specific, nonfunctional routines or rituals
    (3)  stereotyped and repetitive motor mannerisms (e.g., hand or finger flapping or twisting, or complex whole-body movements)
    (4)  persistent preoccupation with parts of objects

C. The disturbance causes clinically significant impairment in social, occupational, or other important areas of functioning.

D. There is no clinically significant general delay in language (e.g., single words used by age 2 years, communicative phrases used by age 3 years).

E. There is no clinically significant delay in cognitive development or in the development of age-appropriate self-help skills, adaptive behavior (other than in social interaction), and curiosity about the environment in childhood.

F. Criteria are not met for another specific Pervasive Developmental Disorder or Schizophrenia.

## Childhood Disintegrative Disorder

A. Apparently normal development for at least the first 2 years after birth as manifested by the presence of age-appropriate verbal and nonverbal communication, social relationships, play, and adaptive behavior.

B. Clinically significant loss of previously acquired skills (before age 10 years) in at least two of the following areas:
   (1) expressive or receptive language
   (2) social skills or adaptive behavior
   (3) bowel or bladder control
   (4) play
   (5) motor skills

C. Abnormalities of functioning in at least two of the following areas:
   (1) qualitative impairment in social interaction (e.g., impairment in nonverbal behaviors, failure to develop peer relationships, lack of social or emotional reciprocity)
   (2) qualitative impairments in communication (e.g., delay or lack of spoken language, inability to initiate or sustain a conversation, stereotyped and repetitive use of language, lack of varied make-believe play)
   (3) restricted, repetitive, and stereotyped patterns of behavior, interests, and activities, including motor stereotypies and mannerisms

D. The disturbance is not better accounted for by another specific Pervasive Developmental Disorder or by Schizophrenia.

## Rett's Disorder

A. All of the following:
   (1) apparently normal prenatal and perinatal development
   (2) apparently normal psychomotor development through the first 5 months after birth
   (3) normal head circumference at birth

B. Onset of all of the following after the period of normal development:
   (1) deceleration of head growth between ages 5 and 48 months
   (2) loss of previously acquired purposeful hand skills between ages 5 and 30 months with the subsequent development of stereotyped hand movements (e.g., hand-wringing or hand washing)
   (3) loss of social engagement early in the course (although often social interaction develops later)
   (4) appearance of poorly coordinated gait or trunk movements
   (5) severely impaired expressive and receptive language development with severe psychomotor retardation

## Pervasive Developmental Disorder Not Otherwise Specified (NOS)

• Disorders with severe developmental deficits not meeting full criteria

## Severity Assessment and Treatment Algorithm

Please refer to Figure 2 for the severity assessment and treatment algorithm for Autism and Pervasive Developmental Disorders.

**Figure 2:** Severity Assessment and Treatment Algorithm for Autism and Pervasive Developmental Disorders

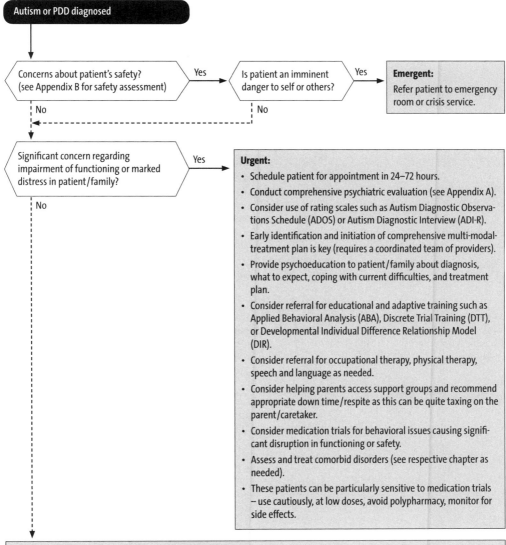

# 14 Delirium

Delirium can be broadly defined as an acute fluctuating global cerebral dysfunction, generally due to a medical condition. The presentation can be quite variable but the core feature is a disturbance in consciousness with a decreased ability to focus, sustain, or shift attention. It is important to note that while many delirious patients may be agitated or obviously suffering from hallucinations; others can appear hypoactive, quiet, and withdrawn. Irritability, mood fluctuation, and anxiety are particularly common findings in pediatric patients suffering from delirium.

In older children and adolescents, the Folstein mini mental status exam (MMSE) can be a useful screen. In younger children who cannot complete the tasks of the MMSE, bedside observation and questioning of parents (or nursing staff if the patient is hospitalized) will be the mainstay of assessment. All patients should be asked whether their thinking is confused and whether they are seeing or hearing any strange things.

## Assessment Algorithm

As only one diagnosis is discussed in this chapter, a diagnostic algorithm is not presented. The only major difference between the different diagnoses is the etiology of the delirium symptoms. Diagnostic criteria are reviewed below and are adapted from the DSM-IV-TR.

## Diagnostic Criteria:

### Delirium Due to General Medical Condition:

- Disturbance of consciousness with reduced ability to focus attention
- A change in memory, disorientation, language disturbance
- Disturbance develops over a period of only hours to days and fluctuates during the course of a day
- There is evidence from a medical evaluation that the disturbance is caused by a medical condition

### Substance-Induced Delirium:

- Substance Intoxication Delirium
  - Disturbance of consciousness with reduced ability to focus attention
  - A change in memory, disorientation, language disturbance
  - Disturbance develops over a period of only hours to days and fluctuates during the course of a day
  - There is evidence from a medical evaluation that the symptoms developed during intoxication from a substance or medication and is the cause of the disturbance
- Substance Withdrawal Delirium
  - Same as above except that medical evaluation shows that the symptoms developed during a withdrawal syndrome and that the symptoms are above and beyond what is expected from withdrawal alone

### Delirium Due to Multiple Etiologies:

- Same as above except that the disturbance has multiple etiologies

### Delirium Not Otherwise Specified:

- When the disturbance does not meet criteria for any of the specific types of delirium mentioned previously

## Severity Assessment and Treatment Algorithm

As delirium is a life-threatening condition, the severity assessment includes only one level, namely emergent. All children and adolescents presenting with delirium should be immediately medically hospitalized for further evaluation and management.

The first priority in the management of delirium is to diagnose and treat any underlying medical cause(s). Often, there are multiple contributing factors, so each should be specifically identified and addressed. Ideally, children with delirium should have a family member or a hospital sitter in their hospital room to provide reassurance and to monitor them for unsafe behaviors.

Mechanical restraints may be required to keep the child from eloping, lashing out at others, or engaging in self-injurious behaviors such as pulling out lines and tubes. Reestablishing normal sleep patterns, ideally through nonpharmacologic interventions, such as discouraging daytime napping and turning off the lights at night, can be extremely helpful as well. Additional environmental interventions include surrounding the patient with pictures of friends and families, treasured items from home (such as a favorite stuffed animal), and a sign/calendar noting the date and the patient's location.

The main pharmacologic interventions for the treatment of delirium are the use of antipsychotic medications while limiting the use of anticholinergic agents and benzodiazepines. Atypical antipsychotic medications such as risperidone, olanzapine, and quetiapine have been used in adults and children as well. However, there is limited data on efficacy and appropriate dosing ranges in pediatric patients for symptoms of delirium. See Chapter 25 for a description of atypical antipsychotic medications.

# 15 Disruptive Behavior Disorders

## Diagnoses Discussed in this Chapter:

- Conduct Disorder
- Oppositional Defiant Disorder
- Disruptive Behavior Disorder Not Otherwise Specified (NOS)

Disruptive behavior disorders are characterized by behaviors that seriously violate the rights of others, violate societal norms, or are antagonistic and defiant. Diagnostic assessment should include an interview with the parent and child, both together and separately. Collecting collateral information from school and probation personnel is also helpful. The interview should include prenatal history, including maternal substance abuse, developmental history, physical and sexual abuse history, and a history of symptom development. Medical history should include history of head trauma, seizures, and chronic illness. Family history must include family coping style, stressors, structure, and limit setting. Academic history should include IQ testing along with history of language, attention, or learning disabilities. Cognitive and educational assessment may need to be performed due to a high association of learning disabilities, borderline intellectual functioning, and mental retardation with conduct disorder. The possibility that disruptive behaviors could be triggered by physical abuse or sexual abuse or neglect should be considered. It is important to assess whether necessary school accommodations are being met to rule out irritable out of control behavior secondary to academic frustration.

## Assessment Algorithm

The assessment algorithm for disruptive behavior disorders is presented in Figure 1. Diagnostic criteria are reviewed below and are adapted from the DSM-IV-TR.

**Figure 1:** Assessment Algorithm for Disruptive Behavior Disorders

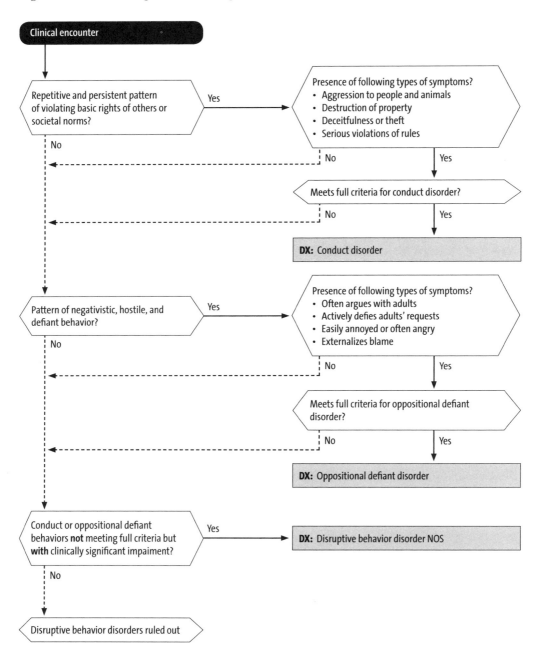

## Diagnostic Criteria

### Conduct Disorder

A. A repetitive and persistent pattern of behavior in which the basic rights of others or major age-appropriate societal norms or rules are violated, as manifested by the presence of three (or more) of the following criteria in the past 12 months, with at least one criterion present in the past 6 months:

**Aggression to people and animals**

(1) often bullies, threatens, or intimidates others
(2) often initiates physical fights
(3) has used a weapon that can cause serious physical harm to others (e.g., a bat, brick, broken bottle, knife, gun)
(4) has been physically cruel to people
(5) has been physically cruel to animals
(6) has stolen while confronting a victim (e.g., mugging, purse snatching, extortion, armed robbery)
(7) has forced someone into sexual activity

**Destruction of property**

(8) has deliberately engaged in fire setting with the intention of causing serious damage
(9) has deliberately destroyed others' property (other than by fire setting)

**Deceitfulness or theft**

(10) has broken into someone else's house, building, or car
(11) often lies to obtain goods or favors or to avoid obligations (i.e., "cons" others)
(12) has stolen items of nontrivial value without confronting a victim (e.g., shoplifting, but without breaking and entering; forgery)

**Serious violations of rules**

(13) often stays out at night despite parental prohibitions, beginning before age 13 years
(14) has run away from home overnight at least twice while living in parental or parental surrogate home (or once without returning for a lengthy period)
(15) is often truant from school, beginning before age 13 years

B. The disturbance in behavior causes clinically significant impairment in social, academic, or occupational functioning.

C. If the individual is age 18 years or older, criteria are not met for Antisocial Personality Disorder.

*Code* based on age at onset:

**312.81   Conduct Disorder, Childhood-Onset Type:** onset of at least one criterion characteristic of Conduct Disorder prior to age 10 years

**312.82   Conduct Disorder, Adolescent-Onset Type:** absence of any criteria characteristic of Conduct Disorder prior to age 10 years

**312.89   Conduct Disorder, Unspecified Onset:** age at onset is not known

*Specify* severity:

**Mild:** few if any conduct problems in excess of those required to make the diagnosis **and** conduct problems cause only minor harm to others

**Moderate:** number of conduct problems and effect on others intermediate between "mild" and "severe"

**Severe:** many conduct problems in excess of those required to make the diagnosis **or** conduct problems cause considerable harm to others

### Oppositional Defiant Disorder

A. A pattern of negativistic, hostile, and defiant behavior lasting at least 6 months, during which four (or more) of the following are present:

    (1)   often loses temper
    (2)   often argues with adults
    (3)   often actively defies or refuses to comply with adults' requests or rules
    (4)   often deliberately annoys people
    (5)   often blames others for his or her mistakes or misbehavior
    (6)   is often touchy or easily annoyed by others
    (7)   is often angry and resentful
    (8)   is often spiteful or vindictive

    **Note:** Consider a criterion met only if the behavior occurs more frequently than is typically observed in individuals of comparable age and developmental level.

B. The disturbance in behavior causes clinically significant impairment in social, academic, or occupational functioning.

C. The behaviors do not occur exclusively during the course of a Psychotic or Mood Disorder.

D. Criteria are not met for Conduct Disorder, and, if the individual is age 18 years or older, criteria are not met for Antisocial Personality Disorder.

### Disruptive Behavior Disorder Not Otherwise Specified (NOS):

- Behaviors or symptoms not meeting criteria for either diagnosis above, but causes functional impairment

The diagnostic criteria for Conduct Disorder and Oppositional Defiant Disorder reprinted with permission from the Diagnostic and Statistical Manual of Mental Disorders, Fourth Edition, Text Revison (© 2000), American Psychiatric Association.

## Severity Assessment and Treatment Algorithm

Please refer to Figure 2 for the severity assessment and treatment algorithm for disruptive behavior disorders

**Figure 2:** Severity Assessment and Treatment Algorithm for Disruptive Behavior Disorders

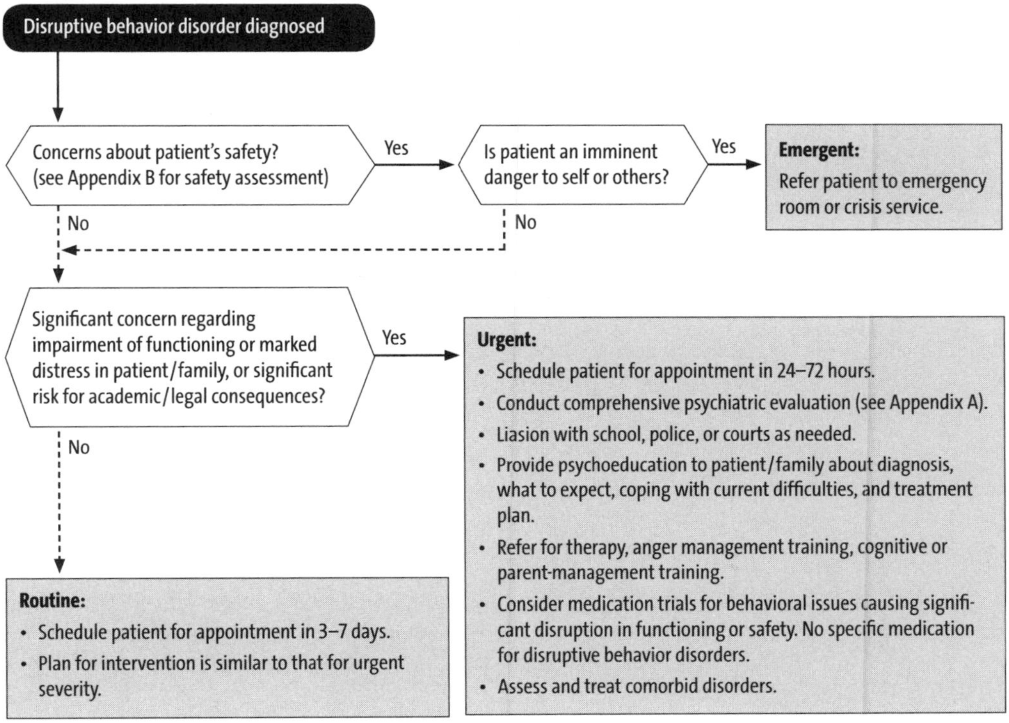

Routine treatment must be multimodal and involve family, school and peer groups. Effective treatment includes multisystemic therapy, parenting skills training, child training in social skills, conflict resolution, and academic skills. Ongoing coordination with school, social services, and juvenile justice personnel is necessary. School interventions may include individualized educational programming and vocational training.

Treatment for school-aged children is more likely to involve school-based interventions, family-based treatment and occasionally individual therapy. In adolescence the emphasis may be more heavily weighted towards individual and family interventions. One of the main parent interventions recommended for younger children is parent management training. The basic components include reducing positive reinforcement of disruptive behavior, increasing reinforcement of prosocial behavior (primarily with parental attention), and applying consequences for disruptive behavior. The pediatrician or PCP can lay the groundwork by providing psychoeducation to the patient and parents, which will hopefully help them get started with the treatment.

Medications are only recommended for treatment of target symptoms and comorbid disorders as medications alone are insufficient treatment for disruptive behavior disorders. Syndromes which may be comorbid or confused with disruptive behavior disorders include Attention Deficit Hyperactivity Disorder, (ADHD), Intermittent Explosive Disorder, Substance Use Disorders, Mood Disorders, Posttraumatic

Stress Disorder, Dissociative Disorders, Seizure Disorder, Pervasive Developmental Disorders, and Mental Retardation. In these cases, disruptive behavioral problems may be secondary to the primary disorder and its treatment may alleviate the behavioral problems. Once the primary diagnosis has been treated, the child must be reevaluated to assess further treatment needs.

# 16 Eating Disorders

## Diagnoses Discussed in this Chapter:

- Anorexia Nervosa
- Bulimia Nervosa
- Eating Disorder Not Otherwise Specificied (NOS)

Eating disorders are diagnosed when the patient is exhibiting symptoms or behaviors that are related to unhappiness with body weight or body image. The two most common disorders that will be encountered are Anorexia Nervosa and Bulimia Nervosa. It is important to note that simply restricting food intake or having binge-eating episodes is not sufficient for either diagnosis. In particular, the presence of purging behaviors can be seen with either diagnosis.

It is important to establish the quantity of weight lost or gained, the period of time over which the change occurred, and the specific patterns of eating behaviors and compensatory behaviors. The patient's perception of his or her body image must be assessed. Finally, physical examination and lab data will help determine the severity of the illness and necessary next steps for stabilization.

## Assessment Algorithm

The assessment algorithm for eating disorders is presented in Figure 1. Diagnostic criteria are reviewed below.

**Figure 1:** Assessment Algorithm for Eating Disorders

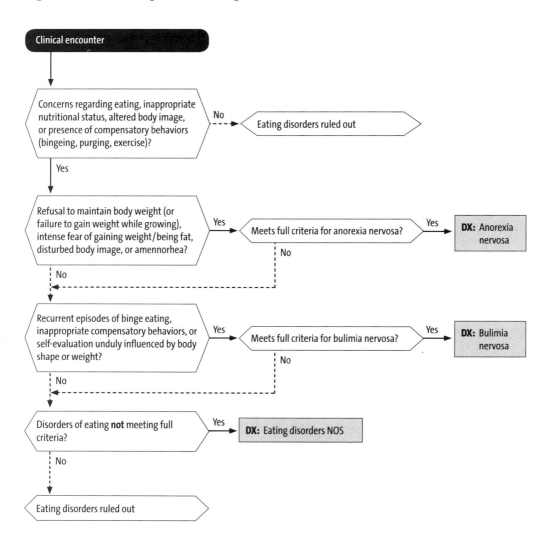

## Diagnostic Criteria

### Anorexia Nervosa

A. Refusal to maintain body weight at or above a minimally normal weight for age and height (e.g., weight loss leading to main-tenance of body weight less than 85% of that expected; or failure to make expected weight gain during period of growth, leading to body weight less than 85% of that expected).
B. Intense fear of gaining weight or becoming fat, even though underweight.
C. Disturbance in the way in which one's body weight or shape is experienced, undue influence of body weight or shape on self-evaluation, or denial of the seriousness of the current low body weight.
D. In postmenarcheal females, amenorrhea, i.e., the absence of at least three consecutive menstrual cycles. (A woman is consid-ered to have amenorrhea if her periods occur only following hormone, e.g., estrogen, administration.)

*Specify* type:

**Restricting Type:** during the current episode of Anorexia Nervosa, the person has not regularly engaged in binge-eating or purging behavior (i.e., self-induced vomiting or the misuse of laxatives, diuretics, or enemas)

**Binge-Eating/Purging Type:** during the current episode of Anorexia Nervosa, the person has regularly engaged in binge-eating or purging behavior (i.e., self-induced vomiting or the misuse of laxatives, diuretics, or enemas)

### Bulimia Nervosa

A. Recurrent episodes of binge eating. An episode of binge eating is characterized by both of the following:
    (1) eating, in a discrete period of time (e.g., within any 2-hour period), an amount of food that is definitely larger than most people would eat during a similar period of time and under similar circumstances
    (2) a sense of lack of control over eating during the episode (e.g., a feeling that one cannot stop eating or control what or how much one is eating)
B. Recurrent inappropriate compensatory behavior in order to prevent weight gain, such as self-induced vomiting; misuse of laxatives, diuretics, enemas, or other medications; fasting; or excessive exercise.
C. The binge eating and inappropriate compensatory behaviors both occur, on average, at least twice a week for 3 months.
D. Self-evaluation is unduly influenced by body shape and weight.
E. The disturbance does not occur exclusively during episodes of Anorexia Nervosa.

*Specify* type:

**Purging Type:** during the current episode of Bulimia Nervosa, the person has regularly engaged in self-induced vomiting or the misuse of laxatives, diuretics, or enemas

**Nonpurging Type:** during the current episode of Bulimia Nervosa, the person has used other inappropriate compensatory behaviors, such as fasting or excessive exercise, but has not regularly engaged in self-induced vomiting or the misuse of laxa-tives, diuretics, or enemas

### Eating Disorder Not Otherwise Specified (NOS):

- Disorders of eating not meeting criteria for any disorder listed above

The diagnostic criteria for Anorexia Nervosa and Bulimia Nervosa reprinted with the permission from the Diagnostic and Statistical Manual of Mental Disorders, Fourth Edition, Text Revison (© 2000), American Psychiatric Association.

## Severity Assessment and Treatment Algorithm

The severity assessment and treatment algorithm for eating disorders is presented in Figure 2.

**Figure 2:** Severity Assessment and Treatment Algorithm for Eating Disorders

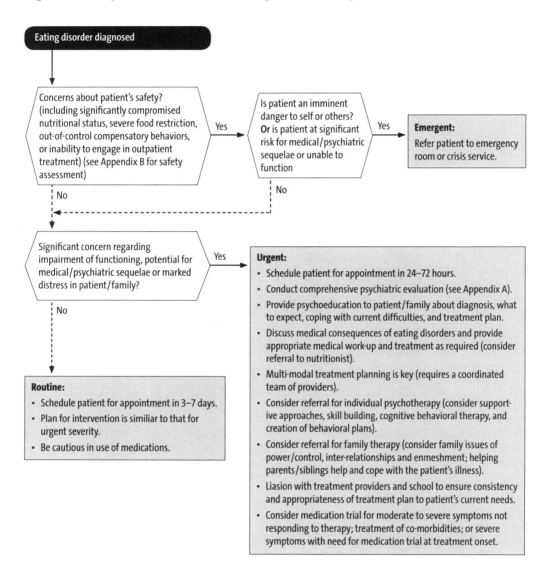

In routine cases, where the patient describes recent onset of symptoms, does not exhibit any physiologic changes, has not lost more than 15% of ideal body weight, and denies any severe psychiatric symptoms; initial management may take place in the primary care setting. If an adolescent medicine or other eating disorder specialist is available, a referral may be considered. These patients will likely require long-term medical follow-up, nutritional education and management, and both individual and family psychotherapy to treat their chronic illness.

Moderate physiologic changes (e.g., mild hypothermia or hypokalemia resolving after oral replacement), weight loss greater than 15% but still less than 20% of ideal body weight, and psychiatric symptoms (e.g., depression) without any acute safety risks may indicate a more **urgent** situation. These patients do not require immediate hospitalization, but should receive a prompt referral to a specialist when available or possibly even to a partial hospitalization program specializing in the treatment of eating disorders. In addition to frequent medical follow-up and extensive education regarding the medical, nutritional, and psychological components to the illness; treatment recommendations include both individual and family therapy to address the behavioral aspects of the dysfunctional eating as well as the parenting implications involved in improving the behaviors. If patients are not able to gain weight consistently on an outpatient basis, they may require a higher level of care. In adults, it has been shown that patients who weigh less than 85% of ideal body weight have an extremely difficult time gaining weight outside an intensively structured program.

Emergent treatment of eating disorders may take two forms, either medical hospitalization for stabilization of physiologic disturbances or psychiatric hospitalization for stabilization of severe psychiatric symptoms, such as suicidality or psychosis. Inpatient medical monitoring is indicated for a weight loss greater than 30% of ideal body weight, vital sign abnormalities (e.g., bradycardia with heart rate <40, hypothermia with temperature <36°C or 96.8°F, hypotension with systolic blood pressure <70, or significant orthostatic hypotension), severe dehydration, severe electrolyte imbalance (including serum potassium <2.5 despite oral replacement, low serum phosphorus, or low serum magnesium), cardiac arrhythmia other than bradycardia, severe binging and purging, or refusal of minimal oral intake (often with associated precipitous weight loss). Correction of fluid and electrolyte status, as well as refeeding in anorexic patients, must occur gradually and in a closely monitored medical environment due to risks such as refeeding syndrome, further electrolyte imbalance, and congestive heart failure. Inpatient or partial hospitalization in a psychiatric facility may be more appropriate in cases when a patient experiences suicidal ideation, psychosis, severe depression, family crisis, or failure to respond to outpatient treatment. For more long-term management of severe eating disorders, residential treatment facilities specializing in eating disorder treatment may be an option.

Psychopharmacological treatment of eating disorders may depend on the specific symptoms of the individual patient and are used regularly to treat comorbid conditions such as depression or anxiety. There is evidence that SSRIs reduce maladaptive eating behaviors in adults with bulimia, but less evidence in terms of the effectiveness of SSRIs and atypical anti-psychotics in anorexia (see Chapter 24 for additional information regarding antidepressant medications and Chapter 25 for additional information regarding atypical antipsychotic medications).

# 17 Learning Disorders

## Diagnoses Discussed in this Chapter:

- Reading Disorder
- Mathematics Disorder
- Disorder of Written Expression
- Learning Disorder Not Otherwise Specified (NOS)

Formerly called Academic Skills Disorders, these disorders affect school performance and can lead to increased frustration, anxiety, acting out, and depression. Early detection, appropriate evaluation, and implementation of treatment with educational support services is key.

## Assessment Algorithm

The assessment algorithm for learning disorders is presented in Figure 1. Diagnostic criteria are reviewed below.

**Figure 1:** Assessment Algorithm for Learning Disorders

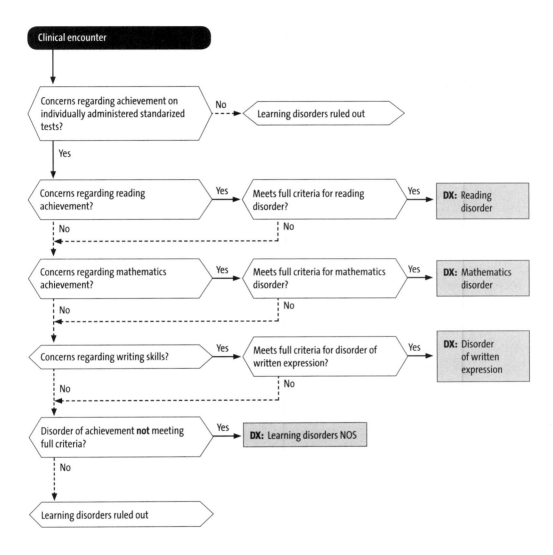

## Diagnostic Criteria

### Reading Disorder

A.  Reading achievement, as measured by individually administered standardized tests of reading accuracy or comprehension, is substantially below that expected given the person's chronological age, measured intelligence, and age-appropriate education.

B.  The disturbance in Criterion A significantly interferes with academic achievement or activities of daily living that require reading skills.

C.  If a sensory deficit is present, the reading difficulties are in excess of those usually associated with it.

**Coding note:** If a general medical (e.g., neurological) condition or sensory deficit is present, code the condition on Axis III.

### Mathematics Disorder

A.  Mathematical ability, as measured by individually administered standardized tests, is substantially below that expected given the person's chronological age, measured intelligence, and age-appropriate education.

B.  The disturbance in Criterion A significantly interferes with academic achievement or activities of daily living that require mathematical ability.

C.  If a sensory deficit is present, the difficulties in mathematical ability are in excess of those usually associated with it.

**Coding note:** If a general medical (e.g., neurological) condition or sensory deficit is present, code the condition on Axis III.

### Disorder of Written Expression

A.  Writing skills, as measured by individually administered standardized tests (or functional assessments of writing skills), are substantially below those expected given the person's chronological age, measured intelligence, and age-appropriate education.

B.  The disturbance in Criterion A significantly interferes with academic achievement or activities of daily living that require the composition of written texts (e.g., writing grammatically correct sentences and organized paragraphs).

C.  If a sensory deficit is present, the difficulties in writing skills are in excess of those usually associated with it.

**Coding note:** If a general medical (e.g., neurological) condition or sensory deficit is present, code the condition on Axis III.

### Learning Disorder Not Otherwise Specified

*   Learning disorders that do not meet full criteria.

The diagnostic criteria for Reading Disorder, Mathematics Disorder, and Disorder of Written Expression reprinted with permission from the Diagnostic and Statistical Manual of Mental Disorders, Fourth Edition, Text Revison (© 2000), American Psychiatric Association.

## Severity Assessment and Treatment Algorithm

A severity assessment and treatment algorithm is not presented for learning disorders as the assessment will not occur in the pediatric or primary care setting. Children suspected of having a learning disorder should be referred for educational, psychological, and/or neuropsychological testing. A major role for the pediatrician or primary care physician lies in early detection of potential problems, monitoring that learning disorders do not impact other aspects of development dramatically, and advocating with parents for appropriate educational services and modifications.

# 18 Mental Retardation

## Diagnosis Discussed in this Chapter:

* Mental Retardation

Mental Retardation is characterized by subaverage intellectual functioning in the context of impairment in adaptive functioning. Psychiatric comorbidity is high in this group of patients. These include ADHD, anxiety disorders, autism and pervasive developmental disorders, and mood disorders. Mental retardation is coded on Axis II.

Treatment options include physical therapy, occupational therapy, educational planning, speech and language therapy, and teaching of self-care and life skills.

## Assessment Algorithm

As only one diagnosis is discussed in this chapter, an assessment algorithm is not presented. Diagnostic criteria are reviewed below.

## Diagnostic Criteria

### Mental Retardation

A. Significantly subaverage intellectual functioning: an IQ of approximately 70 or below on an individually administered IQ test (for infants, a clinical judgment of significantly subaverage intellectual functioning).

B. Concurrent deficits or impairments in present adaptive functioning (i.e., the person's effectiveness in meeting the standards expected for his or her age by his or her cultural group) in at least two of the following areas: communication, self-care, home living, social/interpersonal skills, use of community resources, self-direction, functional academic skills, work, leisure, health, and safety.

C. The onset is before age 18 years.

*Code* based on degree of severity reflecting level of intellectual impairment:

| | | |
|---|---|---|
| 317 | **Mild Mental Retardation:** | IQ level 50–55 to approximately 70 |
| 318.0 | **Moderate Mental Retardation:** | IQ level 35–40 to 50–55 |
| 318.1 | **Severe Mental Retardation:** | IQ level 20–25 to 35–40 |
| 318.2 | **Profound Mental Retardation:** | IQ level below 20 or 25 |
| 319 | **Mental Retardation, Severity Unspecified:** when there is strong presumption of Mental Retardation but the person's intelligence is untestable by standard tests | |

## Severity Assessment and Treatment Algorithm

A severity assessment and treatment algorithm is not presented for mental retardation as the assessment will not occur in the pediatric or primary care setting. After appropriate medical work-up for illnesses affecting cognitive functioning, children suspected of having mental retardation should be referred for educational, psychological, and/or neuropsychological testing. Advocating for appropriate services, referring for occupational/physical therapy, and providing psychoeducation can be invaluable to the child and parents.

# 19 Mood Disorders

## Diagnoses Discussed in this Chapter:

- Bipolar Disorders
  - Bipolar I Disorder
  - Bipolar II Disorder
  - Cyclothymia
  - Bipolar Disorder Not Otherwise Specified NOS
- Depressive Disorders
  - Major Depressive Disorder
  - Dysthymic Disorder
  - Depressive Disorder Not Otherwise Specified NOS
- Mood Disorder Due to General Medical Condition
- Substance-Induced Mood Disorder
- Mood Disorder Not Otherwise Specified (NOS)

Mood disorder symptoms in children and adolescents can vary across developmental stages. Young children usually present with behavioral problems, temper tantrums, somatic complaints, and anxiety symptoms. Older children with mood disorders often describe low self-esteem, hopelessness, and guilt. Adolescents tend to experience changes in sleep and appetite, increased impulsivity or mood lability.

Comorbid anxiety disorders and substance abuse disorders are common and may complicate the clinical picture. Mood disorders are serious and can lead to high-risk behavior, suicidality, self-injurious behavior, or substance abuse. Early detection, proper risk assessment and treatment are paramount.

Please note that Premenstrual Dysphoric Disorder (PMDD) is not covered in this chapter as it is not an official diagnosis in DSM-IV-TR. It is listed under Appendix B of the DSM under "Criteria Sets and Axes Provided for Further Study." Although there are medications that have received FDA approval for the treatment of PMDD (see Chapter 24), it is not a coded DSM diagnosis. In general, patients with PMDD can present with symptoms of depressed mood, hopelessness, self depreciation, anxiety, feeling on edge, affective lability or rejection sensitivity, interpersonal conflicts, decreased interest in usual activities, difficulty concentrating, fatigability, changes in appetite, changes in sleep, feeling overwhelmed or out of control. These patients also present with physical symptoms such as breast tenderness, swelling, bloating, weight gain, or joint or muscle pain.

## Assessment Algorithm

The assessment algorithm for mood disorders is presented in Figure 1. Diagnostic criteria are reviewed below.

**Figure 1:** Assessment Algorithm for Mood Disorders

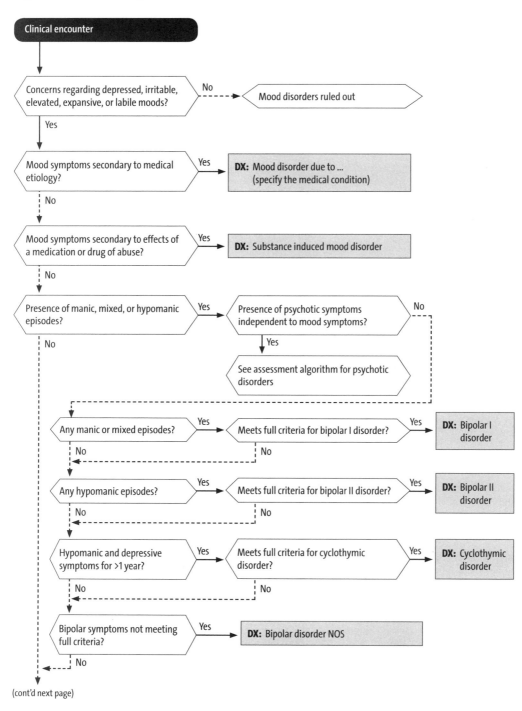

(cont'd next page)

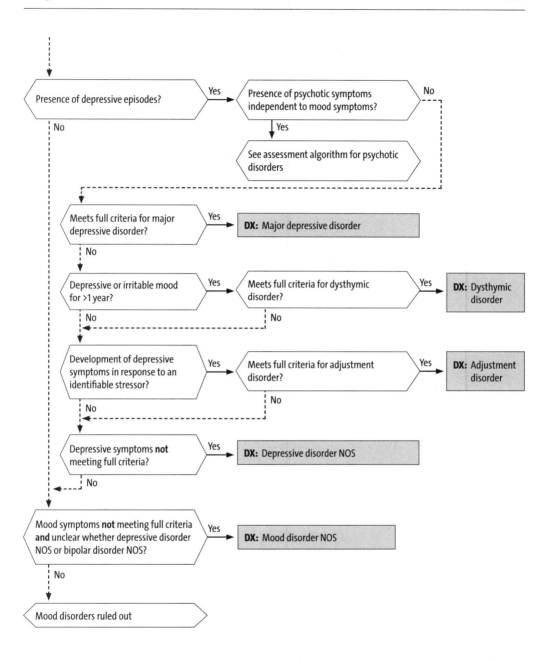

## Diagnostic Criteria

The building blocks for each of the disorders discussed below are mood episodes. Patients may have the presence of one or more separate mood episodes over time. Which mood episodes are present will determine which mood disorder they have.

### Criteria for Manic Episode

A.  A distinct period of abnormally and persistently elevated, expansive, or irritable mood, lasting at least 1 week (or any duration if hospitalization is necessary).

B.  During the period of mood disturbance, three (or more) of the following symptoms have persisted (four if the mood is only irritable) and have been present to a significant degree:

  (1)  inflated self-esteem or grandiosity
  (2)  decreased need for sleep (e.g., feels rested after only 3 hours of sleep)
  (3)  more talkative than usual or pressure to keep talking
  (4)  flight of ideas or subjective experience that thoughts are racing
  (5)  distractibility (i.e., attention too easily drawn to unimportant or irrelevant external stimuli)
  (6)  increase in goal-directed activity (either socially, at work or school, or sexually) or psychomotor agitation
  (7)  excessive involvement in pleasurable activities that have a high potential for painful consequences (e.g., engaging in unrestrained buying sprees, sexual indiscretions, or foolish business investments)

C.  The symptoms do not meet criteria for a Mixed Episode (see below).

D.  The mood disturbance is sufficiently severe to cause marked impairment in occupational functioning or in usual social activities or relationships with others, or to necessitate hospitalization to prevent harm to self or others, or there are psychotic features.

E.  The symptoms are not due to the direct physiological effects of a substance (e.g., a drug of abuse, a medication, or other treatment) or a general medical condition (e.g., hyperthyroidism).

  **Note:**  Manic-like episodes that are clearly caused by somatic antidepressant treatment (e.g., medication, electroconvulsive therapy, light therapy) should not count toward a diagnosis of Bipolar I Disorder.

### Criteria for Hypomanic Episode

A.  A distinct period of persistently elevated, expansive, or irritable mood, lasting throughout at least 4 days, that is clearly different from the usual nondepressed mood.

B.  During the period of mood disturbance, three (or more) of the following symptoms have persisted (four if the mood is only irritable) and have been present to a significant degree:

  (1)  inflated self-esteem or grandiosity
  (2)  decreased need for sleep (e.g., feels rested after only 3 hours of sleep)
  (3)  more talkative than usual or pressure to keep talking
  (4)  flight of ideas or subjective experience that thoughts are racing
  (5)  distractibility (i.e., attention too easily drawn to unimportant or irrelevant external stimuli)
  (6)  increase in goal-directed activity (either socially, at work or school, or sexually) or psychomotor agitation
  (7)  excessive involvement in pleasurable activities that have a high potential for painful consequences (e.g., the person engages in unrestrained buying sprees, sexual indiscretions, or foolish business investments)

C.  The episode is associated with an unequivocal change in functioning that is uncharacteristic of the person when not symptomatic.

D.  The disturbance in mood and the change in functioning are observable by others.

E.  The episode is not severe enough to cause marked impairment in social or occupational functioning, or to necessitate hospitalization, and there are no psychotic features.

F.  The symptoms are not due to the direct physiological effects of a substance (e.g., a drug of abuse, a medication, or other treatment) or a general medical condition (e.g., hyperthyroidism).

    **Note:** Hypomanic-like episodes that are clearly caused by somatic antidepressant treatment (e.g., medication, electroconvulsive therapy, light therapy) should not count toward a diagnosis of Bipolar II Disorder.

## Criteria for Major Depressive Episode

A.  Five (or more) of the following symptoms have been present during the same 2-week period and represent a change from previous functioning; at least one of the symptoms is either (1) depressed mood or (2) loss of interest or pleasure.

    **Note:** Do not include symptoms that are clearly due to a general medical condition, or mood-incongruent delusions or hallucinations.

    (1) depressed mood most of the day, nearly every day, as indicated by either subjective report (e.g., feels sad or empty) or observation made by others (e.g., appears tearful). **Note:** In children and adolescents, can be irritable mood.
    (2) markedly diminished interest or pleasure in all, or almost all, activities most of the day, nearly every day (as indicated by either subjective account or observation made by others)
    (3) significant weight loss when not dieting or weight gain (e.g., a change of more than 5% of body weight in a month), or decrease or increase in appetite nearly every day. **Note:** In children, consider failure to make expected weight gains.
    (4) insomnia or hypersomnia nearly every day
    (5) psychomotor agitation or retardation nearly every day (observable by others, not merely subjective feelings of restlessness or being slowed down)
    (6) fatigue or loss of energy nearly every day
    (7) feelings of worthlessness or excessive or inappropriate guilt (which may be delusional) nearly every day (not merely self-reproach or guilt about being sick)
    (8) diminished ability to think or concentrate, or indecisiveness, nearly every day (either by subjective account or as observed by others)
    (9) recurrent thoughts of death (not just fear of dying), recurrent suicidal ideation without a specific plan, or a suicide attempt or a specific plan for committing suicide

B.  The symptoms do not meet criteria for a Mixed Episode (see p. 365).

C.  The symptoms cause clinically significant distress or impairment in social, occupational, or other important areas of functioning.

D.  The symptoms are not due to the direct physiological effects of a substance (e.g., a drug of abuse, a medication) or a general medical condition (e.g., hypothyroidism).

E.  The symptoms are not better accounted for by Bereavement, i.e., after the loss of a loved one, the symptoms persist for longer than 2 months or are characterized by marked functional impairment, morbid preoccupation with worthlessness, suicidal ideation, psychotic symptoms, or psychomotor retardation.

## Criteria for Mixed Episode

A.  The criteria are met both for a Manic Episode (see above) and for a Major Depressive Episode (see above) (except for duration) nearly every day during at least a 1-week period.

B.  The mood disturbance is sufficiently severe to cause marked impairment in occupational functioning or in usual social activities or relationships with others, or to necessitate hospitalization to prevent harm to self or others, or there are psychotic features.

C.  The symptoms are not due to the direct physiological effects of a substance (e.g., a drug of abuse, a medication, or other treatment) or a general medical condition (e.g., hyperthyroidism).

    **Note:** Mixed-like episodes that are clearly caused by somatic antidepressant treatment (e.g., medication, electroconvulsive therapy, light therapy) should not count toward a diagnosis of Bipolar I Disorder.

## Bipolar Mood Disorders

These disorders are characterized by fluctuating mood states. There may be *Manic, Hypomanic, or Major Depressive episodes* present.

- Bipolar I Disorder:
    - At least one *Manic* or *Mixed* episode
    - There may be *Hypomanic* or *Major Depressive* episodes as well
    - There is significant distress and functioning is impaired

- Bipolar II Disorder:
    - Presence or history of at least one *Major Depressive* episode
    - Presence or history of at least one *Hypomanic* episode
    - There has never been a *Manic* or *Mixed* episode
    - There is significant distress and functioning is impaired

- Cyclothymic Disorder:
    - For at least one year (two years in adults), there have been many periods with hypomanic symptoms and many periods with depressive symptoms that do not meet criteria for a *Major Depressive* episode
    - During that one year, the patient has not been symptom free for more than two months at a time
    - No *Major Depressive, Manic , or Mixed* episode has been present during the first 1 year of illness
    - The symptoms are not due to the direct effect of a substance or of a medical condition
    - There is significant distress and impairment in daily functioning
- Bipolar Disorder NOS:
    - Bipolar features are present but criteria are not met for any specific bipolar disorder

## Depressive Mood Disorders

These are characterized by depressed mood states. There is no evidence of *Manic, Hypomanic, or Mixed episodes*.

- Major Depressive Disorder:
    - Presence of at least one *Major Depressive* episode.
    - There is significant distress and impaired daily functioning

- Dysthymic Disorder:
    - Depressed (or irritable in children and adolescents) mood for most of the day, for more days than not, either by patient report or by the observation of others, for at least one year (two years in adults)
    - Presence, while depressed, of two of the following:
        - Poor appetite or overeating
        - Insomnia or hypersomnia
        - Low energy or fatigue
        - Low self-esteem
        - Trouble concentrating or difficulty in making decisions
        - Feelings of hopelessness
    - During the one year period, the patient has not been without symptoms for more than two months at a time
    - No *Major Depressive* episode has been present during the first year of the disturbance
    - There has never been a *Manic, Mixed, or Hypomanic* episode
    - There is significant distress and impaired daily functioning

- Depressive Disorder NOS:
  - A disorder with depressive features that does not meet criteria for another depressive disorder or adjustment disorder
- Mood Disorder Due to General Medical Condition:
  - Presence of mood symptoms
  - Disturbance is due to direct physiological consequence of a general medical condition
- Substance-Induced Mood Disorder:
  - Presence of mood symptoms
  - Disturbance is due to effects of a substance or medication
- Mood Disorder Not Otherwise Specified (NOS):
  - Mood symptoms are present but do not meet criteria for any specific disorder listed above

The diagnostic criteria for Manic Episode, Hypomanic Episode, Major Depressive Episode, and Mixed Episode reprinted with permission from the Diagnostic and Statistical Manual of Mental Disorders, Fourth Edition, Text Revison (© 2000), American Psychiatric Association.

## Severity Assessment and Treatment Algorithm

Please see Figure 2 for the severity assessment and treatment algorithm for mood disorders.

**Figure 2:** Severity Assessment and Treatment Algorithm for Mood Disorders

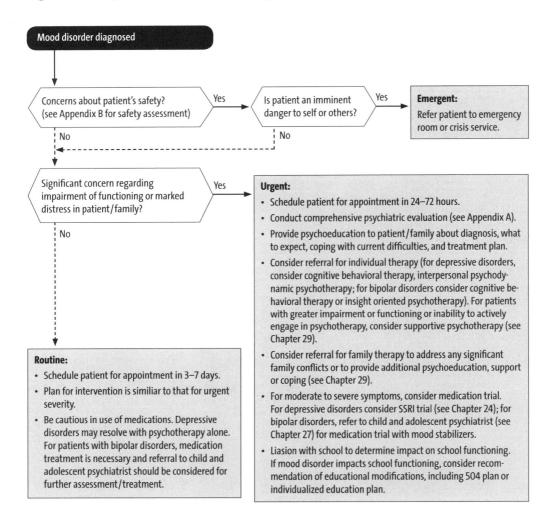

# 20 Psychotic Disorders

## Diagnoses Discussed in this Chapter:

- Brief Psychotic Disorder
- Delusional Disorder
- Schizoaffective Disorder
- Schizophreniform Disorder
- Schizophrenia
- Shared Psychotic Disorder
- Psychotic Disorder Due to General Medical Condition
- Substance Induced Psychotic Disorder
- Psychotic Disorder Not Otherwise Specified (NOS)

While significantly less common than other diagnoses, psychotic disorders are important to recognize and diagnose. Patients with a newly diagnosed psychotic disorder (i.e., first-break psychosis) or prominent psychotic symptoms should be referred to a child and adolescent psychiatrist. Due to the severity of psychotic disorders and psychotic symptoms in regards to implications for psychopathology, routine follow-up and treatment should only occur in direct consultation with a child and adolescent psychiatrist. In areas where one may not be available, appropriate assessment and treatment requires the input of a physician (i.e., a psychiatrist). Patients who are stable and are on an appropriate medication regimen may be managed by the pediatrician or PCP.

## Assessment Algorithm

The assessment algorithm for psychotic disorders is presented in Figure 1. Diagnostic criteria are reviewed below.

**Figure 1: Assessment Algorithm for Psychotic Disorders**

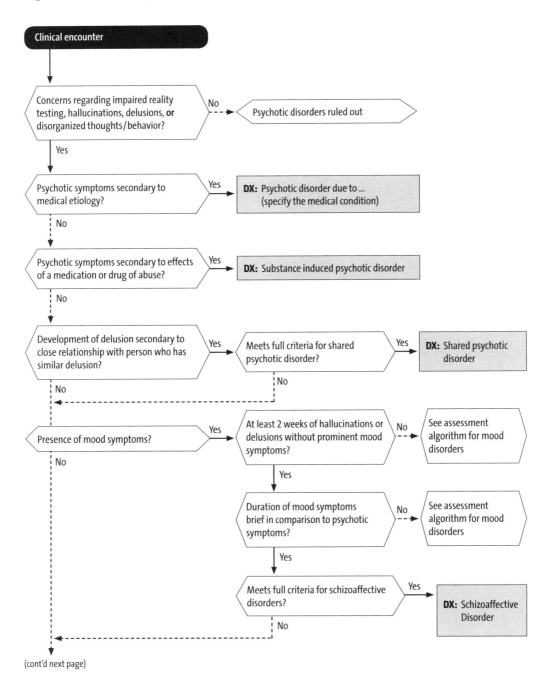

(cont'd next page)

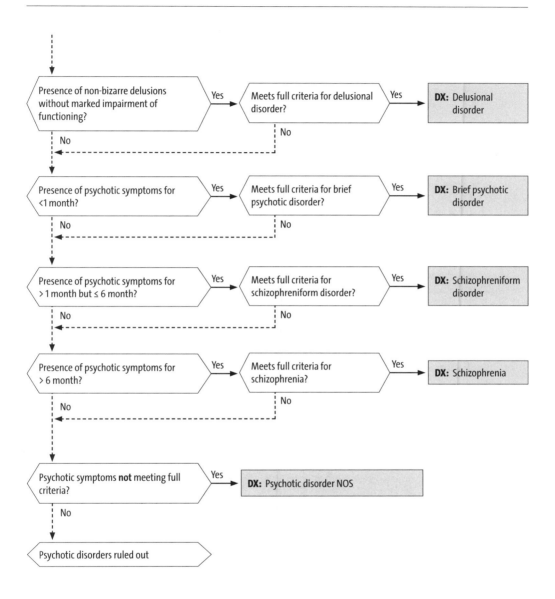

Presence of non-bizarre delusions without marked impairment of functioning? — Yes → Meets full criteria for delusional disorder? — Yes → **DX:** Delusional disorder

No → Meets full criteria for delusional disorder? — No

Presence of psychotic symptoms for <1 month? — Yes → Meets full criteria for brief psychotic disorder? — Yes → **DX:** Brief psychotic disorder

No → Meets full criteria for brief psychotic disorder? — No

Presence of psychotic symptoms for >1 month but ≤ 6 month? — Yes → Meets full criteria for schizophreniform disorder? — Yes → **DX:** Schizophreniform disorder

No → Meets full criteria for schizophreniform disorder? — No

Presence of psychotic symptoms for >6 month? — Yes → Meets full criteria for schizophrenia? — Yes → **DX:** Schizophrenia

No → Meets full criteria for schizophrenia? — No

Psychotic symptoms **not** meeting full criteria? — Yes → **DX:** Psychotic disorder NOS

No

Psychotic disorders ruled out

## Diagnostic Criteria

### Brief Psychotic Disorder

A. Presence of one (or more) of the following symptoms:
   (1)  delusions
   (2)  hallucinations
   (3)  disorganized speech (e.g., frequent derailment or incoherence)
   (4)  grossly disorganized or catatonic behavior
   **Note:** Do not include a symptom if it is a culturally sanctioned response pattern.

B. Duration of an episode of the disturbance is at least 1 day but less than 1 month, with eventual full return to premorbid level of functioning.

C. The disturbance is not better accounted for by a Mood Disorder With Psychotic Features, Schizoaffective Disorder, or Schizophrenia and is not due to the direct physiological effects of a substance (e.g., a drug of abuse, a medication) or a general medical condition.

*Specify* if:

**With Marked Stressor(s)** (brief reactive psychosis):  if symptoms occur shortly after and apparently in response to events that, singly or together, would be markedly stressful to almost anyone in similar circumstances in the person's culture

**Without Marked Stressor(s):**   if psychotic symptoms do **not** occur shortly after, or are not apparently in response to events that, singly or together, would be markedly stressful to almost anyone in similar circumstances in the person's culture

**With Postpartum Onset:**  if onset within 4 weeks postpartum

### Delusional Disorder

A. Nonbizarre delusions (i.e., involving situations that occur in real life, such as being followed, poisoned, infected, loved at a distance, or deceived by spouse or lover, or having a disease) of at least 1 month's duration.

B. Criterion A for Schizophrenia has never been met. **Note:** Tactile and olfactory hallucinations may be present in Delusional Disorder if they are related to the delusional theme.

C. Apart from the impact of the delusion(s) or its ramifications, functioning is not markedly impaired and behavior is not obviously odd or bizarre.

D. If mood episodes have occurred concurrently with delusions, their total duration has been brief relative to the duration of the delusional periods.

E. The disturbance is not due to the direct physiological effects of a substance (e.g., a drug of abuse, a medication) or a general medical condition.

*Specify* type (the following types are assigned based on the predominant delusional theme):

**Erotomanic Type:**  delusions that another person, usually of higher status, is in love with the individual

**Grandiose Type:**   delusions of inflated worth, power, knowledge, identity, or special relationship to a deity or famous person

**Jealous Type:**  delusions that the individual's sexual partner is unfaithful

**Persecutory Type:**  delusions that the person (or someone to whom the person is close) is being malevolently treated in some way

**Somatic Type:**  delusions that the person has some physical defect or general medical condition

**Mixed Type:**  delusions characteristic of more than one of the above types but no one theme predominates

**Unspecified Type**

## Schizoaffective Disorder

A. An uninterrupted period of illness during which, at some time, there is either a Major Depressive Episode, a Manic Episode, or a Mixed Episode concurrent with symptoms that meet Criterion A for Schizophrenia.

**Note:** The Major Depressive Episode must include Criterion A1: depressed mood.

B. During the same period of illness, there have been delusions or hallucinations for at least 2 weeks in the absence of prominent mood symptoms.

C. Symptoms that meet criteria for a mood episode are present for a substantial portion of the total duration of the active and residual periods of the illness.

D. The disturbance is not due to the direct physiological effects of a substance (e.g., a drug of abuse, a medication) or a general medical condition.

*Specify* type:

**Bipolar Type:** if the disturbance includes a Manic or a Mixed Episode (or a Manic or a Mixed Episode and Major Depressive Episodes)

**Depressive Type:** if the disturbance only includes Major Depressive Episodes

## Schizophreniform Disorder:

- Patient has symptoms of Schizophrenia
- Duration at least one month but not more than six months

## Schizophrenia

A. *Characteristic symptoms:* Two (or more) of the following, each present for a significant portion of time during a 1-month period (or less if successfully treated):

(1) delusions
(2) hallucinations
(3) disorganized speech (e.g., frequent derailment or incoherence)
(4) grossly disorganized or catatonic behavior
(5) negative symptoms, i.e., affective flattening, alogia, or avolition

**Note:** Only one Criterion A symptom is required if delusions are bizarre or hallucinations consist of a voice keeping up a running commentary on the person's behavior or thoughts, or two or more voices conversing with each other.

B. *Social/occupational dysfunction:* For a significant portion of the time since the onset of the disturbance, one or more major areas of functioning such as work, interpersonal relations, or self-care are markedly below the level achieved prior to the onset (or when the onset is in childhood or adolescence, failure to achieve expected level of interpersonal, academic, or occupational achievement).

C. *Duration:* Continuous signs of the disturbance persist for at least 6 months. This 6-month period must include at least 1 month of symptoms (or less if successfully treated) that meet Criterion A (i.e., active-phase symptoms) and may include periods of prodromal or residual symptoms. During these prodromal or residual periods, the signs of the disturbance may be manifested by only negative symptoms or two or more symptoms listed in Criterion A present in an attenuated form (e.g., odd beliefs, unusual perceptual experiences).

D. *Schizoaffective and Mood Disorder exclusion:* Schizoaffective Disorder and Mood Disorder With Psychotic Features have been ruled out because either (1) no Major Depressive, Manic, or Mixed Episodes have occurred concurrently with the active-phase symptoms; or (2) if mood episodes have occurred during active-phase symptoms, their total duration has been brief relative to the duration of the active and residual periods.

E. *Substance/general medical condition exclusion:* The disturbance is not due to the direct physiological effects of a substance (e.g., a drug of abuse, a medication) or a general medical condition.

F.  *Relationship to a Pervasive Developmental Disorder:* If there is a history of Autistic Disorder or another Pervasive Developmental Disorder, the additional diagnosis of Schizophrenia is made only if prominent delusions or hallucinations are also present for at least a month (or less if successfully treated).

*Classification of longitudinal course* (can be applied only after at least 1 year has elapsed since the initial onset of active-phase symptoms):

**Episodic With Interepisode Residual Symptoms** (episodes are defined by the reemergence of prominent psychotic symptoms); also specify if: **With Prominent Negative Symptoms**

**Episodic With No Interepisode Residual Symptoms**

**Continuous** (prominent psychotic symptoms are present throughout the period of observation); also *specify if:* **With Prominent Negative Symptoms**

**Single Episode In Partial Remission**; also *specify if:* **With Prominent Negative Symptoms**

**Single Episode In Full Remission**

**Other or Unspecified Pattern**

### Shared Psychotic Disorder:

*   The delusion develops in the context of a close relationship with another person
*   It is similar to the other person's delusion

### Psychotic Disorder Due to General Medical Condition:

*   Presence of hallucinations or delusions
*   Symptoms are due to a general medical condition

### Substance-Induced Psychotic Disorder:

*   Presence of hallucinations or delusions
*   Symptoms are due to a substance or medication

### Psychotic Disorder Not Otherwise Specified (NOS):

*   Psychotic symptoms not meeting criteria for any of the diagnoses listed above

The diagnostic criteria for Brief Psycotic Disorder, Delusional Disorder, Schizoaffective Disorder, and Schizophrenia reprinted with permission from the Diagnostic and Statistical Manual of Mental Disorders, Fourth Edition, Text Revison (© 2000), American Psychiatric Association.

## Severity Assessment and Treatment Algorithm

Please see Figure 2 for the severity assessment and treatment algorithm for psychotic disorders.

**Figure 2: Severity Assessment and Treatment Algorithm for Psychotic Disorders**

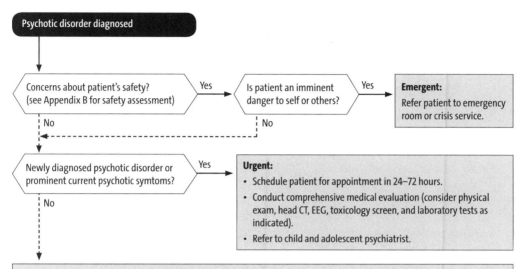

**Routine:**

- Schedule patient for appointment in 3–7 days.
- Continue to monitor patient's psychotic symptoms and response to treatment
- Due to the severity of psychotic disorders and psychotic symptoms, routine follow-up and treatment should only occur in direct consultation with a child and adolescent psychiatrist. Appropriate assessment and on-going comprehensive treatment requires input of physician (i.e., a psychiatrist).
- Patients on antipsychotic medication should be routinely monitored for metabolic syndrome and medication-induced extrapyramidal symptoms of movement disorders. Consider routine use of Abnormal Involuntary Movement Scale (AIMS) and Simpson Angus Scale (SAS).

# 21 Somatoform and Factitious Disorders

Somatoform disorders involve physical complaints which cannot be fully explained by a known general medical condition or the direct effects of a substance. Somatoform disorders are typically diagnoses of exclusion and almost always warrant medical work-up.

Factitious disorders are considered when the patient is intentionally producing symptoms to assume the sick role. In factitious disorder by proxy, which is coded as a Factitious Disorder NOS, a person produces these symptoms in another such as a parent producing symptoms in a child. Patients presenting with malingering produce symptoms for a secondary gain such as financial compensation. Please note that malingering is a V-code diagnosis which is coded on Axis I.

## Assessment Algorithm

The assessment algorithm for somatoform disorders is presented in Figure 1. Factitious disorders and malingering are included in Figure 1 to aid to simplifying the diagnostic process. Please note that factitious disorders and malingering are not subcategories of somatoform disorder in DSM-IV-TR. Diagnostic criteria are reviewed below.

**Figure 1:** Assessment Algorithm for Somatoform Disorders

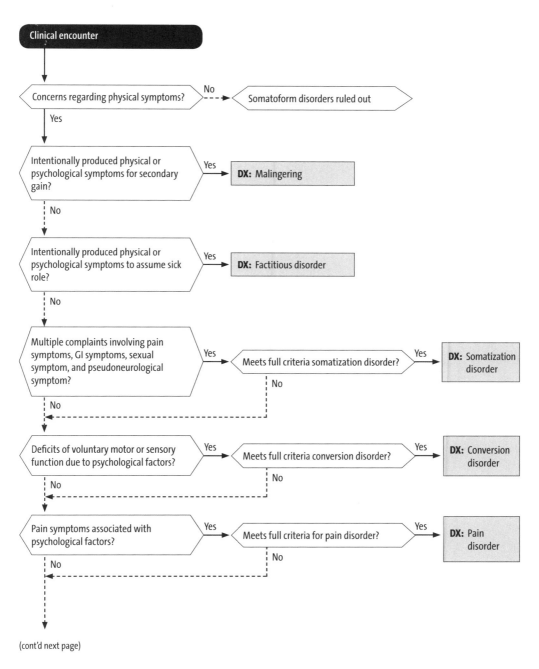

(cont'd next page)

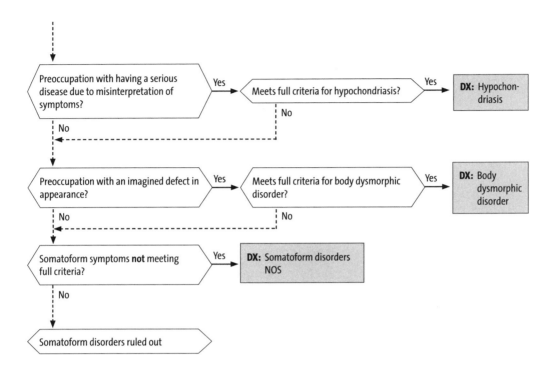

## Diagnostic Criteria

### Body Dysmorphic Disorder:

- Preoccupation with an imagined defect in appearance, or excessive concern over a slight physical anomaly
- The preoccupation causes impairment in functioning or significant distress

### Conversion Disorder:

- There are one or more symptoms/deficits affecting sensory function or motor function that suggest a neurological or other medical condition
- The onset of the symptoms and/or exacerbation of symptoms is preceded by a conflict/stressor
- The symptom/deficit is not intentionally produced and cannot be fully explained by a medical condition
- Specify whether the type of symptom or deficit is:
  - Motor
  - Sensory
  - Seizures
  - Mixed

### Hypochondriasis:

- Preoccupation with fear of having a serious disease
- This continues despite medical workup and reassurance
- The belief is not delusional in severity
- The duration is at least six months
- Specify whether with poor insight

### Pain Disorder:

- Pain in one or more sites
- Psychological factors play an important role
- The pain is not intentional or feigned

### Somatization Disorder:

- A history of multiple physical complaints beginning before age 30 years
- These physical complaints include each of the following:
  - Four pain symptoms
  - Two gastrointestinal symptoms
  - One sexual symptom
  - One pseudoneurological symptom (not pain)
- The symptoms cannot be fully explained by a known medical condition or the symptoms are in excess of what would be expected
- The symptoms are not intentionally produced

**Somatization Disorder Not Otherwise Specified (NOS):**

- Somatoform symptoms not meeting criteria for a specific disorder above

**Factitious Disorder:**

- Producing or feigning of symptoms
- Done to assume sick role

**Factitious Disorder Not Otherwise Specified (NOS):**

- Factitious symptoms not meeting full criteria for factitious disorder

**Malingering:**

- Intentionally producing false or exaggerated symptoms for external rewards

## Severity Assessment and Treatment Algorithm

Somatization disorders, factitious disorders, and malingering do present in pediatric and primary care settings. A key factor to consider is whether the presentation is placing the child at risk. Specifically, is the child's physical or emotional integrity being compromised due to any of these disorders? Is the patient being exposed to unnecessary medical tests or procedures? Is the parent or guardian causing physical or psychological harm for an ulterior motive? Principles of evaluating for child abuse and neglect should be the initial intervention.

Once safety has been determined, appropriate medical evaluation is necessary to rule out physical symptoms due to a general medical condition. Once the patient has been ruled out for a medical condition, consideration should be given for referral to a specialist.

A severity assessment and treatment algorithm is not presented as the steps likely to occur in the pediatric or primary care setting involve routine medical decision making.

These patients may be reluctant to see their symptoms as being anything but physiologically based, so a close collaboration between the pediatrician or PCP and the mental health provider is key. In order to manage the patient's or guardian's ability to manage these symptoms, consider setting regular appointments to limit exacerbations and urgent care visits to your practice or the emergency room. Obtaining consultation with a specialist is necessary as these patients can be influenced by a wide range of psychological stressors and motives. It is important to create a treatment plan that does not estrange or disenfranchise the patient or guardian while having them obtain necessary treatment.

# 22 Substance Use Disorders

**Diagnoses Discussed in this Chapter:**

- Substance Intoxication
- Substance Abuse
- Substance Dependence
- Substance Withdrawal

Children and adolescents who abuse substances often present with significant changes in mood, cognition, and behavior. Behavioral changes include agitation, irritability, hyperactivity, disinhibition, out-of-control behavior, and hypervigilance. To be considered a disorder, the substance must produce impairment in psychiatric, behavioral, family, academic, recreational, or medical domains. Screening should include assessment for interpersonal impairment, academic decline, and familial dysfunction. Contributions to substance abuse in adolescents include genetic predisposition, peer pressure, and efforts to alleviate depression, anxiety, stress, or disturbing emotions.

Toxicology screening is recommended when abuse is suspected, keeping in mind the detection periods for commonly abused drugs (see Figure 1).

**Figure 1:** Detection Periods for Commonly Abused Drugs

| Urine Toxicology | Detection after last use |
|---|---|
| Amphetamines | 1–2 days |
| Barbiturates | 3–14 days |
| Benzodiazepines | 2–9 days |
| Cocaine | 2–4 days |
| Methaqualone | 7–14 days |
| Opiates | 1–2 days |
| Phencyclidine | 2–8 days |
| Cannabinoids | 2–8 days (acute) 14–42 days (chronic) |

Substances not typically included in standard urine toxicology screens include LSD, psilocybin, MDMA, MDA, as well as other designer drugs. Be aware for signs of inhalant abuse including spots or sores around the mouth, injected eyes, rhinorrhea, dizziness, nausea, or loss of appetite.

Initial assessment should include determining the quantity and frequency of use for each substance. Consider using a standard screening tool such as the CRAFFT (see Figure 2). Gathering information from a variety of sources, including parents, patient, school, involved social agencies, and previous treatment records, may provide more accurate and comprehensive reporting of current substance use and resultant functioning.

Screening for comorbid psychiatric disorders is essential as many adolescents referred for substance abuse treatment may also require treatment for ADHD, Oppositional Defiant Disorder, Conduct Disorder, Depression, Anxiety Disorder, or PTSD. Adolescents may be self medicating a preexisting undiagnosed psychiatric disorder or the symptoms may be a consequence of the substance abuse. When attempting to diagnose a comorbid psychiatric disorder, it is important to establish the presence of symptoms during extended periods of sobriety from abused substances.

**Figure 2:** CRAFFT Substance Abuse Screening Test

| | |
|---|---|
| **C**ar | Have you ever ridden in a car driven by someone (including yourself) who was high or had been using alcohol or drugs? |
| **R**elax | Do you ever use alcohol or drugs to relax, feel better about yourself, or fit in? |
| **A**lone | Do you ever use alcohol or drugs while you are by yourself or alone? |
| **F**orget | Do you ever forget things that you did while using alcohol or drugs? |
| **F**amily | Do your family or friends ever tell you that you should cut down on your drinking or drug use? |
| **T**rouble | Have you ever gotten into trouble while you were using alcohol or drugs? |

Scoring: Two or more positive responses indicate the need for further assessment.

Adapted from: Knight JR, Sherritt L, Shrier LA, Harris SK, & Chang G. Validity of the CRAFFT substance abuse screening test among adolescent clinic patients. *Arch Pediatr Adolesc Med.* 2002; *156*(6):607–614.

## Assessment Algorithm

Figure 3 presents intoxication and withdrawal syndromes for substances of abuse.

## Diagnostic Criteria

### Substance Intoxication:

- Developing a syndrome of reversible symptoms after ingestion of a substance
- There are maladaptive behavioral or psychological changes

### Substance Abuse

A. A maladaptive pattern of substance use leading to clinically significant impairment or distress, as manifested by one (or more) of the following, occurring within a 12-month period:

(1) recurrent substance use resulting in a failure to fulfill major role obligations at work, school, or home (e.g., repeated absences or poor work performance related to substance use; substance-related absences, suspensions, or expulsions from school; neglect of children or household)

(2) recurrent substance use in situations in which it is physically hazardous (e.g., driving an automobile or operating a machine when impaired by substance use)

(3) recurrent substance-related legal problems (e.g., arrests for substance-related disorderly conduct)

(4) continued substance use despite having persistent or recurrent social or interpersonal problems caused or exacerbated by the effects of the substance (e.g., arguments with spouse about consequences of intoxication, physical fights)

B. The symptoms have never met the criteria for Substance Dependence for this class of substance.

## Substance Dependence

A maladaptive pattern of substance use, leading to clinically significant impairment or distress, as manifested by three (or more) of the following, occurring at any time in the same 12-month period:

1) tolerance, as defined by either of the following:
   (a) a need for markedly increased amounts of the substance to achieve intoxication or desired effect
   (b) markedly diminished effect with continued use of the same amount of the substance

(2) withdrawal, as manifested by either of the following:
   (a) the characteristic withdrawal syndrome for the substance (refer to Criteria A and B of the criteria sets for Withdrawal from the specific substances)
   (b) the same (or a closely related) substance is taken to relieve or avoid withdrawal symptoms

(3) the substance is often taken in larger amounts or over a longer period than was intended

(4) there is a persistent desire or unsuccessful efforts to cut down or control substance use

(5) a great deal of time is spent in activities necessary to obtain the substance (e.g., visiting multiple doctors or driving long distances), use the substance (e.g., chain-smoking), or recover from its effects

(6) important social, occupational, or recreational activities are given up or reduced because of substance use

(7) the substance use is continued despite knowledge of having a persistent or recurrent physical or psychological problem that is likely to have been caused or exacerbated by the substance (e.g., current cocaine use despite recognition of cocaine-induced depression, or continued drinking despite recognition that an ulcer was made worse by alcohol consumption)

*Specify* if:

**With Physiological Dependence:** evidence of tolerance or withdrawal (i.e., either item 1 or 2 is present)

**Without Physiological Dependence:** no evidence of tolerance or withdrawal (i.e., neither item 1 nor 2 is present)

*Course specifiers* (see text for definitions):

**Early Full Remission**

**Early Partial Remission**

**Sustained Full RemissionSustained Partial Remission**

**On Agonist Therapy**

**In a Controlled Environment**

## Substance Withdrawal:

- Developing a syndrome of symptoms after cessation or reduction in use of a substance
- This causes a significant impairment in functioning.

The diagnostic criteria for Substance Abuse and Substance Dependence reprinted with permission from the Diagnostic and Statistical Manual of Mental Disorders, Fourth Edition, Text Revison (© 2000), American Psychiatric Association.

**Figure 3:** Intoxication and Withdrawal Syndromes for Substances of Abuse

|  | Intoxication | Withdrawal |
|---|---|---|
| **Alcohol** | – Slurred speech<br>– Incoordination<br>– Unsteady gait<br>– Nystagmus<br>– Impaired attention or memory<br>– Stupor/coma | – Autonomic hyperactivity<br>– Increased hand tremor<br>– Insomnia<br>– Nausea or vomiting<br>– Transient visual, tactical, or auditory hallucinations<br>– Psychomotor agitation<br>– Anxiety<br>– Grand mal seizures |
| **Amphetamine** | – Tachycardia or bradycardia<br>– Pupillary dilation<br>– Elevated or lowered blood pressure<br>– Perspiration or chills<br>– Nausea or vomiting<br>– Psychomotor agitation or retardation<br>– Weight loss<br>– Muscle weakness, respiratory depression, chest pain or cardiac arrhythmias | – Dysphoric mood<br>– Fatigue<br>– Vivid, unpleasant dreams<br>– Insomnia or hypersomnia<br>– Increased appetite<br>– Psychomotor agitation or retardation |
| **Caffeine (>250mg)** | – Restlessness<br>– GI disturbance<br>– Nervousness<br>– Muscle twitching<br>– Excitement<br>– Tachycardia<br>– Insomnia<br>– Inexhaustibility<br>– Flushed face<br>– Psychomotor agitation<br>– Diuresis<br>– Rambling thoughts or speech | None |
| **Cannabis** | – Symptoms within 2 hours<br>– Conjunctival injection<br>– Increased appetite<br>– Dry mouth<br>– Tachycardia | None |
| **Cocaine** | – Tachycardia or bradycardia<br>– Pupillary dilation<br>– Elevated or lowered blood pressure<br>– Perspiration or chills<br>– Nausea or vomiting<br>– Psychomotor agitation or retardation<br>– Weight loss<br>– Muscle weakness, respiratory depression, chest pain or cardiac arrhythmias | – Dysphoric mood<br>– Fatigue<br>– Vivid, unpleasant dreams<br>– Insomnia or hypersomnia<br>– Increased appetite<br>– Psychomotor agitation or retardation |

**Figure 3:** Continued

|  | Intoxication | Withdrawal |
|---|---|---|
| **Hallucinogen** | – Tachycardia<br>– Pupillary dilation<br>– Sweating<br>– Palpitations<br>– Blurred vision<br>– Tremors<br>– Incoordination | None |
| **Inhalant** | – Dizziness<br>– Nystagmus<br>– Incoordination<br>– Slurred speech<br>– Unsteady gait<br>– Lethargy<br>– Depressed reflexes<br>– Psychomotor retardation<br>– Tremor<br>– Blurred vision or diplopia<br>– Stupor or coma | None |
| **Nicotine** | None | – Dysphoric or depressed mood<br>– Insomnia<br>– Irritability, frustration, or anger<br>– Anxiety<br>– Increased appetite or weight gain<br>– Difficulty concentrating<br>– Restlessness<br>– Decreased heart rate |
| **Opioids** | – Drowsiness or coma<br>– Slurred speech<br>– Impaired attention or memory | – Dysphoric mood<br>– Nausea or vomiting<br>– Muscle aches<br>– Lacrimation or rhinnorhea<br>– Diarrhea<br>– Yawning<br>– Pupillary dilation, piloerection, or sweating<br>– Fever<br>– Insomnia |
| **Phencyclidine** | – Vertical or horizontal nystagmus<br>– Hypertension or tachycardia<br>– Decreased response to pain<br>– Ataxia<br>– Dysarthria<br>– Muscle rigidity<br>– Seizures<br>– Hyperacusis | None |

**Figure 3:** Continued

| | Intoxication | Withdrawal |
|---|---|---|
| **Sedative, Hypnotic, or Anxiolytic** | – Slurred speech<br>– Incoordination<br>– Unsteady gait<br>– Nystagmus<br>– Impaired attention or memory<br>– Stupor or coma | – Autonomic hyperactivity<br>– Increased hand tremor<br>– Insomnia<br>– Nausea or vomiting<br>– Transient visual, tactical, or auditory hallucinations<br>– Psychomotor Agitation<br>– Anxiety<br>– Grand mal seizures |

## Severity Assessment and Treatment Algorithm

A severity assessment and treatment algorithm is not presented as many substances are presented. Despite multiple substances of abuse, treatment options are few and described below. Once substance use has been determined by history and/or toxicology screen, severity must be assessed in terms of frequency, nature, and amount of use. The youth's attitude towards use, associated changes in functioning, and related risky behaviors should be discussed. Many adolescents exhibit mild substance abuse problems due to curiosity or experimentation, with occasional alcohol or marijuana use resulting in little or no change in behaviors or mood.

Routine management may consist of anticipatory guidance, education, and recommendations for drug-free alternatives. More regular use of alcohol or marijuana, using other substances, use during the school week, and use that affects mood and school performance or attendance may indicate a more moderate substance abuse problem. These children and families may require more urgent management, including a psychiatric referral, individual or family therapy, group therapy in the context of a drug-free self-help group, and ongoing monitoring in the office possibly with periodic drug screening. Finally, in severe cases, the daily use of illicit, prescription, or over-the-counter drugs may lead to psychological and/or chemical dependency, significant mood symptoms, school failure, family conflict, and legal difficulties. These patients will likely require separation from the drugs and peer group more emergently, with either short-term psychiatric hospitalization or placement in a residential treatment facility. Occasionally, medical hospitalization or acute detoxification may be required first. Upon discharge, these adolescents and families will require intensive outpatient monitoring, preferably from a multi-disciplinary treatment team.

Pharmacologic treatment may play a role in treatment as it does in adults, especially in those patients with additional comorbid psychiatric diagnoses. In adults, evidence-based psychosocial treatments for substance use disorders include cognitive-behavioral therapies (e.g., relapse prevention, social skills training), motivational enhancement therapy (MET), behavioral therapies (e.g., community reinforcement, contingency management), 12-step facilitation (e.g., Alcoholics or Narcotics Anonymous), psychodynamic therapy, interpersonal therapy, self-help manuals, behavioral self-control, brief interventions, case management, and group, marital, and family therapies.

# Section IV
# Toolbox of Interventions

This section presents information related to treatment options for psychiatric illnesses. The treatments are subdivided into biological interventions, psychotherapeutic interventions, and psychosocial interventions. Each chapter provides a *Treatment Description* and *Clinical Pearls* to maximize treatment compliance and efficacy while limiting potential side effects. As certain interventions require description beyond the scope of this text, Appendix F provides *References and Sources for Additional Information* to guide the user to trusted sources regarding the use of that intervention.

As you become more familiar with these treatments, you may find yourself significantly impacting the lives of the youths you treat. If so, please let us know.

**This section reviews the following treatments:**

- Alpha Adrenergic Agonists
- Antidepressants
- Atypical Antipsychotics
- Benzodiazepines
- Mood Stabilizers and Lithium
- Stimulants and Related ADHD Medications
- Planning for Psychotherapeutic Interventions
- Planning for Psychosocial Supports

# Pharmacological Interventions

# 23 Alpha Adrenergic Agonists

Clonidine and guanfacine are alpha adrenergic agonist medications that are prescribed off label for the management of ADHD symptoms and impulsivity. They may also be useful for the management of tics and sleep difficulties. They are also used for their mild anti-anxiety effects.

These medications may be considered for the management of ADHD in cases where the parents request a nonstimulant medication or in patients who have failed multiple stimulant trials as well as atomoxetine. Stimulants are the first line medications for ADHD.

They are both generally well tolerated, but should be titrated and tapered cautiously due to effects on blood pressure. Guanfacine is associated with less sedation than clonidine. Please refer to the individual descriptions below for additional information.

## Clonidine (Catapres; Catapres Transdermal Therapeutic System)

### Treatment Description

#### FDA Approved Uses:

- Clonidine is a centrally acting alpha-agonist that is FDA approved for the treatment of hypertension. It is not FDA approved for the treatment of any psychiatric disorders. Its safety and efficacy has not been established in children under the age of 12.

#### Off-Label Uses:

- Clonidine is also used for the management of ADHD, impulsivity, and aggression. It is also used as a sleeping aid and to manage tics. These are off-label uses of the medication and are not FDA approved.

#### Black Box Warnings:

- None

## Dosage Forms:

- Tablets: 0.1 mg, 0.2 mg, 0.3 mg.

- Transdermal (once-weekly) patch: 0.1 mg/24 h, 0.2 mg/24 h, and 0.3 mg/24 h.

## Dosing on Initiation:

- Initial dose of 0.05 mg/day; increase every 3–7 days by 0.05 mg/day to a maximum of 3–5 mcg/kg/day given in divided doses three times a day (maximum dose is 0.3–0.4 mg/day).

## Dosing on Discontinuation:

- If the drug needs to be discontinued, gradually taper the dose over a week as abrupt discontinuation has the potential for a rapid increase in blood pressure.

- Sudden cessation of clonidine treatment has, in some cases, resulted in symptoms such as nervousness, agitation, headache, and tremor accompanied or followed by a rapid rise in blood pressure and elevated catecholamine concentrations in the plasma.

- Rare instances of hypertensive encephalopathy, cerebrovascular accidents, and death have been reported in adults after clonidine withdrawal.

- An excessive rise in blood pressure following abrupt discontinuation of clonidine can be treated with oral clonidine or intravenous phentolamine.

- If the patient is taking a beta-blocker and clonidine, the beta-blocker should be discontinued several days before starting the taper off clonidine.

## Side Effects:

- The most common side effects are sedation, dizziness (most likely from hypotension), dry mouth, and constipation. Skin irritation can occur with use of the transdermal patch.

- Many children will develop tolerance to the sedation over the course of a few weeks.

- Youths who may be driving or engaging in potentially hazardous activities should be counseled about its sedative effects. They should know that using alcohol, barbiturates, or other sedating drugs may worsen these effects.

- Monitor pulse and blood pressure. Consider ECG monitoring if clinically indicated or if used in combination with other medications which affect cardiac functioning.

## Contraindications:

- Known hypersensitivity to clonidine.

- Clonidine should be used cautiously in patients with severe coronary insufficiency, conduction disturbances, recent myocardial infarction, cerebrovascular disease, or chronic renal failure.

## Drug-Drug Interactions:

- Significant interactions are reviewed below. Before selecting any specific medication, please be sure to reference the current prescribing information from the manufacturer for that specific drug for additional information.

- Clonidine may potentiate the CNS-depressive effects of alcohol, barbiturates, or other sedating drugs.

- Avoid use with tricyclic antidepressants as this may lead to increased blood pressure.

- Avoid use with beta-blockers as this may potentiate bradycardia.

### Clinical Pearls

- Consider use of clonidine in patients with ADHD symptoms, impulsivity, or aggression with a comorbid tic disorder. Stimulant medications can exacerbate tics, thus making clonidine a good option.

- Consider use of clonidine with Autism and Pervasive Developmental Disordered youths with hyperarousal.

- Tends to be effective as a sleep aide, but proper sleep hygiene and behavioral interventions should be attempted first.

- Can be used to decrease hyperarousal in patients with PTSD as well as for mild anxiety symptoms. However, SSRI medications are the first line of treatment for anxiety disorders, including PTSD.

- When initiating clonidine, begin with a bedtime dose as the most common side effect is sedation. It is also helpful to have parents first administer the medication over the weekend, so that they can be familiar with its effects on their child. Likewise, the school nurse should be notified that the child is taking this medication.

- It is helpful to keep teachers in the loop about a new medication trial as well. They can provide valuable information regarding the child's response to the medication in the classroom setting and around peers. Also, in case the child has any side-effects, they can alert the school nurse and parents.

- There is some concern that Clonidine may worsen depressive symptoms, so monitor for their onset and be sure to ask about family history.

- For some children in whom oral clonidine has stopped working, switching to the transdermal patch may be helpful. However, if a patient has had an allergic reaction to the transdermal patch, some may also have difficulty with the oral form.

- Please use caution if prescribing clonidine and stimulants in combination. Although no link has been made, there are case reports about sudden deaths in children taking this combination. It is advised that the prescribing physician review current data at the time of consideration, obtain appropriate informed consent, and consider frequent monitoring for potential side effects.

## Guanfacine (Tenex)

### Treatment Description

#### FDA Approved Uses:

- Guanfacine is a centrally acting alpha 2 agonist that is FDA approved for the treatment of hypertension. It is not FDA approved for the treatment of any psychiatric disorders. Its safety and efficacy has not been established in children under the age of 12.

#### Off-Label Uses

- Guanfacine is also used for the management of ADHD and impulsivity. It may also be used as a sleeping aid and to manage tics. These are off-label uses of the medication and are not FDA approved.

#### Black Box Warnings:

- None

#### Dosage Forms:

- Tablets: 1 mg, 2 mg

#### Dosing on Initiation:

- Start at 0.25 mg bid, increase by 0.5 mg per day weekly as tolerated (maximum 45 micrograms/kg/day or 4 mg/day). It is longer acting than clonidine and can be dosed bid.

#### Dosing on Discontinuation:

- If the drug needs to be discontinued, gradually taper the dose over as abrupt discontinuation has the potential for a rapid increase in blood pressure.
- Sudden cessation of guanfacine treatment has, in some cases, resulted in symptoms such as nervousness, anxiety, and rebound hypertension.
- Rebound hypertension generally occurs 2–4 days after abrupt withdrawal due to the long half life of guanfacine. Blood pressure slowly returns to pretreatment levels in 2 to 4 days.
- If the patient is taking a beta-blocker and guanfacine, the beta-blocker should be discontinued several days before starting to taper off guanfacine.

#### Side Effects:

- The most common side effects are dry mouth, sedation, weakness, dizziness, constipation, and impotence. Most are experienced as mild and may improve on continued dosing.
- Youths who may be driving or engaging in potentially hazardous activities should be counseled about its sedative effects. They should know that using alcohol, barbiturates, or other sedating drugs may worsen these effects.

- They should also be warned that their tolerance for alcohol and other CNS depressants may be diminished.

### Contraindications:

- It should not be used in patients with known hypersensitivity to guanfacine.

- Guanfacine should be used cautiously in patients with severe coronary insufficiency, recent myocardial infarction, cerebrovascular disease, or chronic renal or hepatic failure.

### Drug-Drug Interactions:

- Significant interactions are reviewed below. Before selecting any specific medication, please be sure to reference the current prescribing information from the manufacturer for that specific drug for additional information.

- Guanfacine may potentiate the CNS-depressive effects of alcohol, barbiturates or other sedating drugs.

- Avoid use with tricyclic antidepressants as this may lead to increased blood pressure.

- Avoid use with beta-blockers as this may potentiate bradycardia.

## Clinical Pearls

- Guanfacine may be more helpful for inattentive symptoms than clonidine with less sedation.

- Consider use of guanfacine with Autism and Pervasive Developmental Disordered youths with hyperactivity and inattention.

- Can be used to decrease nightmares in patients with PTSD as well as for mild anxiety symptoms. However, SSRI medications are the first line of treatment for anxiety disorders, including PTSD.

- When initiating guanfacine, begin with a bedtime dose as sedation is a common side effect. It is also helpful to have parents first administer the medication over the weekend, so that they can be familiar with its effects on their child. Likewise, the school nurse should be notified that the child is taking this medication.

- It is helpful to keep teachers in the loop about a new medication trial as well. They can provide valuable information regarding the child's response to the medication in the classroom setting and around peers. Also, in case the child has any side-effects, they can alert the school nurse and parents.

- There is some concern that guanfacine may be associated with mania and aggressive behavioral changes in pediatric patients with ADHD. These case reports all had medical or family risk factors for bipolar disorder. All patients recovered upon discontinuation of guanfacine HCl.

# 24 Antidepressants

## Medications Discussed in this Chapter:

- Fluoxetine
- Sertraline
- Citalopram
- Escitalopram
- Fluvoxamine
- Bupropion
- Mirtazapine
- Venlafaxine

Selective serotonin reuptake inhibitors (SSRI) antidepressants are the medication of choice for the treatment of childhood anxiety and depressive disorders. They are generally well tolerated with mild or transient side effects including headaches, gastrointestinal distress and insomnia.

Before prescribing SSRIs, carefully assess for the possibility of symptoms of bipolar disorder as SSRIs may result in worsening of such symptoms or may trigger a manic episode. It is also important to carefully discuss the FDA black box warning regarding worsening of suicidal thinking.

Non-SSRI antidepressant medications are listed due to their common use (see Table 1 for a comparison of antidepressants). A patient should receive at least 2 adequate SSRI antidepressant trials prior to considering other classes. Also, should the patient experience side effects, possible switching to hypomania or mania, or worsening of symptoms – referral to a child and adolescent psychiatrist should be considered for reevaluation of the diagnosis as well as further treatment.

**Table 1: Comparison of antidepressant medications**

| Generic Name | Brand Name | Dosages (mg) | FDA Approval |
|---|---|---|---|
| *Selective Serotonin Reuptake Inhibitors (SSRIs)* | | | |
| Fluoxetine ⚠ | Prozac Sarafem | Oral solution: 20 mg/5 ml Tablets: 10 mg (scored) 10, 20 mg Prozac capsules: 10, 20, 40 mg Sarafem capsules: 10, 20 mg | Depression in children 8–17 years of age as well as adults Obsessive compulsive disorder (OCD) in children 7–17 years of age as well as adults |

**Table 1:** Continued

| Generic Name | Brand Name | Dosages (mg) | FDA Approval |
|---|---|---|---|
| | | Start at 5mg to 10 mg PO daily, titrate in 10 mg increments. Max. dose in adults is 60 mg daily. | Binge-eating and vomiting behaviors in adults with moderate to severe bulimia nervosa<br><br>Panic disorder, with or without agoraphobia, in adults |
| Sertraline ⚠ | Zoloft | Oral solution (concentrate): 20 mg/ml<br>Tablets: 25, 50, 100 mg<br><br>Start at 25mg PO daily, titrate in 25 mg increments. Max. dose in adults is 200 mg daily. | OCD in children 6–17 years of age as well as in adults<br><br>Depression in adults<br><br>Panic disorder, with or without agoraphobia, in adults<br><br>Posttraumatic stress disorder in adults<br><br>Premenstrual dysphoric disorder (PMDD) in adults<br><br>Social anxiety disorder in adults |
| Citalopram ⚠ | Celexa | Oral solution: 10 mg/5 ml<br>Tablets: 10, 20, 40 mg<br><br>Start at 10 mg PO daily, titrate in 10 mg increments. Max. dose in adults is 60 mg daily. | Depression in adults |
| Escitalopram ⚠ | Lexapro | Oral solution: 1 mg/ml<br>Tablets: 5, 10, 20 mg<br><br>Start at 5mg PO daily, titrate in 5mg increments. Max. dose in adults is 20 mg daily. | Depression in adults<br><br>Generalized anxiety disorder in adults |
| Fluvoxamine ⚠ | Luvox | Tablets: 25, 50, 100 mg<br><br>Start at 50 mg PO daily, titrate in 25 mg increments. Max. dose in adolescents is 200 mg daily. Dose may be divided qd or bid. | OCD in children 8–17 years of age as well as in adults |

**Table 1:** Continued

| Generic Name | Brand Name | Dosages (mg) | FDA Approval |
|---|---|---|---|
| *Non-SSRI Antidepressants* | | | |
| Buproprion ⚠ | Wellbutrin Wellbutrin SR, Wellbrutrin XL | Tablets: 75, 100 mg (begin at bid, go to tid) Tablets (SR): 100, 150, 200 mg (needs to be given bid) Tablets (XL): 150, 300 mg (used qd)  Start at 1.4 mg/kd/day, titrate in 37.5 mg increments. Max. dose in adolescents is 6 mg/kg/day up to 450 mg/day. Dose may be divided qd or bid depending on formulation. | Depression in adults |
| Mirtazapine ⚠ | Remeron Remeron SolTab | Tablets: 15, 30, 45 mg Tablets, orally-disintegrating (all contain phenylalanine): 15, 30, 45 mg  Start at 7.5mg PO daily, titrate in 7.5 mg increments. Max. dose in adults is 45 mg daily.  Better to take medication at bedtime due to sedation. | Depression in adults |
| Venlafaxine ⚠ | Effexor Effexor XR | Tablets: 25, 37.5, 50, 75, 100 Capsules (XR): 37.5, 75, 150 mg  Start at 37.5 mg, increase in 37.5 mg increments. Max. dose in adults is 375 mg daily. Divide daily dose bid or tid. | Depression in adults  Generalized anxiety disorder in adults  Social anxiety disorder in adults  Panic disorder, with or without agoraphobia, in adults |

⚠ Please see the Black Box Warning in the Treatment Description section.

## Treatment Description:

### FDA Approved Uses:

- Please see Table 1.

### Off-Label Uses:

- The above listed medications are used off-label for the treatment of depression, premenstrual dysphoric disorder, generalized anxiety disorder, panic disorder, obsessive compulsive disorder, social anxiety disorder, posttraumatic stress disorder, and bulimia nervosa. Patients should begin with trials of SSRI antidepressants before moving onto other classes.

- They are also used for the treatment of separation anxiety disorder and selective mutism.

- Bupropion is used for attention deficit hyperactivity disorder (ADHD), particularly in teens with substance use disorders where concern may exist about prescribing stimulants.

- Bupropion is also used for patients who have experienced sexual side effects on other agents, but need treatment for mood and anxiety disorders.

- Mirtazapine is used in children and adolescents who are depressed and have significant insomnia or poor appetite.

- These are off-label uses of these medications and are not FDA approved.

 **Black Box Warning**
**Suicidality and Antidepressant Drugs**

Antidepressants increased the risk compared to placebo of suicidal thinking and behavior (suicidality) in children, adolescents, and young adults in short-term studies of major depressive disorder (MDD) and other psychiatric disorders. Anyone considering the use of any antidepressant in a child, adolescent, or young adult must balance this risk with the clinical need. Short-term studies did not show an increase in the risk of suicidality with antidepressants compared to placebo in adults beyond age 24; there was a reduction in risk with antidepressants compared to placebo in adults aged 65 and older. Depression and certain other psychiatric disorders are themselves associated with increases in the risk of suicide. Patients of all ages who are started on antidepressant therapy should be monitored appropriately and observed closely for clinical worsening, suicidality, or unusual changes in behavior. Families and caregivers should be advised of the need for close observation and communication with the prescriber.

The FDA has recommended weekly monitoring for the first 4 weeks after initiating an antidepressant medication followed by every other week for the next 4 weeks. When the dosage is stabilized, the patient should be assessed every three months. Once the patient has had a remission of symptoms, the medication should be continued for at least 9 months to prevent relapse.

## Dosage Forms:

- Please see Table 1.

## Dosing on Initiation:

- Commonly used SSRIs for children include fluoxetine and sertraline. A medication trial of fluoxetine should include an initial dose of 5–10 mg daily for seven days and if tolerated, dosage should be increased by 10 mg on the second week. Doses typically range from 5–60 mg/day based upon clinical response. Some patients with significant anxiety or poor sleep find fluoxetine difficult to tolerate. If using fluoxetine for these patients, start at a lower dose and titrate slowly. If the patient has a worsening of anxiety or sleep, consider using a different antidepressant.

- A trial of sertraline should begin with doses of 25 mg with an increase to 50 mg if tolerated after seven days. Sertraline may be considered for patients who have significant anxiety symptoms or sleep difficulties as it is better tolerated by such patients. Doses typically range from 25 to 200 mg/day based upon clinical response.

- The duration of an adequate trial of an SSRI is four to six weeks at the appropriate dose. In general, there is a fine balance between keeping patients on the lowest dose possible and getting them to the appropriate dose quickly. Start at the lowest dose for one week to assess for tolerability. As a general rule, this should be about half the normal starting dose for adults or about a quarter for children. The dose can then be increased on the second week. From this point, the patient should be assessed for response to that particular dose. If no change in symptoms has occurred after 2 to 3 weeks at a given dose, consider titrating to a higher dose. If you begin to see an improvement in symptoms, wait to see the full effects of that dose for 4 to 6 weeks.

- If a maximal dose is reached without adequate therapeutic effect or if further dosage increases are limited by medication side effects, switching to another antidepressant is indicated.

## Dosing on Discontinuation:

- Antidepressant medications should be gradually tapered to avoid any withdrawal side effects.

- Fluoxetine has a long half-life and can be quickly discontinued as it has limited withdrawal side effects. However, due to its long half-life, there must be a proper drug washout before starting another antidepressant due to the possibility of serotonin syndrome.

## Side Effects:

- Gastrointestinal (GI) intolerance can be common including nausea, vomiting, and dyspepsia. These side effects do worsen with more rapid dose titrations. Depending on the medication, it may either cause decreased appetite or weight gain.

- Insomnia, sedation, increased nightmares, and decreased REM sleep may be experienced depending on the medication.

    - Agitation, irritability, restlessness, and activation can also be seen. Increased anxiety, panic attacks, hostility, aggression, impulsivity, psychomotor restlessness, hypomania, and mania are also possible.

    - Sexual dysfunction is seen with SSRI medications as well as with non-SSRI agents. Bupropion has a more favorable sexual side effect profile.

  - Hyponatremia, serotonin syndrome, and cardiovascular side effects can also occur.
  - Emergence of worsening depression, hypomania, mania, or increased suicidal thoughts should be monitored for.
- Please check the prescribing information for the medication that you are considering for specific side-effect details.

## Contraindications:

- Known hypersensitivity to the medication.
- Please check the prescribing information for the medication that you are considering for specific contraindications.

## Drug-Drug Interactions:

- Many drug-drug interactions can occur when using antidepressant medications. Please check the prescribing information for the medication that you are considering for specific information regarding drug-drug interactions.

## Clinical Pearls

- Use with caution and start at very low dose in children with family history of mood disorder, especially bipolar disorder, as these agents can cause activation in susceptible children and adolescents.
- Start with very low dose if treating children on the autism spectrum.

# 25 Atypical Antipsychotics

**Medications Discussed in this Chapter:**

- Aripiprazole
- Olanzapine
- Quetiapine
- Risperidone
- Ziprasidone

Atypical antipsychotic medications can be effective treatments for psychosis, mood episodes, agitation, and movement disorders (see Table 1 for a comparison of atypical antipsychotic medications). Though initially touted for their favorable side-effect profiles, significant concerns exist regarding their potential for metabolic syndrome and other serious side effects.

In discussing antipsychotic medications, older classes of medication have been excluded from this text. The diagnosis and treatment of psychotic disorders, as well as bipolar disorder are, in our professional opinion, reaching the edges of what can be safely and effectively managed by the pediatrician or PCP without consultation of a specialist. This information is provided for those who feel comfortable with prescribing and managing atypical antipsychotic medications. As previously discussed in the chapter on psychotic disorders, patients with a newly diagnosed psychotic disorder (i.e., first break psychosis) or prominent psychotic symptoms should be referred to a child and adolescent psychiatrist. Due to the severity of psychotic disorders and psychotic symptoms in regards to implications for psychopathology, routine follow-up and treatment should only occur in direct consultation with a child and adolescent psychiatrist. In areas where one may not be available, appropriate assessment and treatment requires the input of a physician (i.e., a psychiatrist). Patients who are stable and are on an appropriate medication regimen may be managed by the pediatrician or PCP.

For the assessment and treatment of bipolar disorder or mixed mood episodes, similarly, consider referral to a child and adolescent psychiatrist. Patients who are stable and are on an appropriate medication regimen may be managed by the pediatrician or PCP.

**Table 1:**   Comparison of Atypical Antipsychotic Agents

| Generic Name | Brand Name | Dosages (mg) | FDA Approvals |
|---|---|---|---|
| Aripiprazole ⚠[1] ⚠[2] | Abilify | Tablets: 2, 5, 10, 15, 20, 30 mg<br>Oral Disintegrating Tablets: 10, 15<br>Oral Solution: 1 mg/mL<br>IM Injection<br><br>Start at 2 mg daily for 2 days; increase to 5 mg daily for 2 days; then increase in 5 mg increments as clinically indicated. Max. 30 mg/day in adolescents. | Acute and maintenance treatment of Schizophrenia in adults and adolescents aged 13–17 years<br><br>Acute and maintenance treatment of manic and mixed episodes of Bipolar I in adults and patients aged 10–17 years<br><br>Adjunctive therapy to lithium or valproate for acute and maintenance treatment of manic and mixed episodes of Bipolar I in adults and patients aged 10–17 years<br><br>Adjunctive therapy to antidepressants for the acute treatment of Major Depressive Disorder in adults<br><br>Injection is indicated for the acute treatment of agitation associated with Schizophrenia or Bipolar Disorder, manic or mixed in adults |
| Olanzapine ⚠[2] | Zyprexa | Tablets: 2.5, 5, 7.5, 15, 20 mg<br>Oral Disintegrating Tablets: 5, 10, 15, 20 mg<br>IM Injection<br><br>Start at 2.5 mg to 5 mg, increase weekly in 5 mg increments as clinically indicated. Max. 20 mg/day in adults. | Schizophrenia in adults<br><br>Manic and mixed episodes of Bipolar I in adults<br><br>Combination therapy with lithium or valproate for treatment of manic and mixed episodes of Bipolar I in adults<br><br>Injection is indicated for the acute treatment of agitation associated with Schizophrenia or Bipolar Disorder, manic or mixed in adults |

**Table 1:** Continued

| Generic Name | Brand Name | Dosages (mg) | FDA Approvals |
|---|---|---|---|
| Quetiapine ⚠️¹ ⚠️² | Seroquel | Tablets: 25, 50, 100, 200, 300, 400 mg<br><br>Start at 12.5 mg to 25 mg daily, increase in 25 mg to 50 mg increments as clinically indicated. Divide daily dose to administer for bid or tid dosing. Max. 800 mg/day in adults. | Bipolar depression in adults<br><br>Acute manic episodes of Bipolar I as monotherapy or as adjunct to lithium or divalproex in adults<br><br>Maintenance treatment of Bipolar I as adjunct to lithium or divalproex in adults<br><br>Schizophrenia in adults |
| Risperidone ⚠️² | Risperdal | Tablets: 0.25, 0.5, 1, 2, 3, 4 mg<br>Oral Disintegrating Tablets: 0.5,1,2,3,4 mg<br>IM Injection<br><br>Start at 0.25 mg to 0.5 mg daily for 4 days, then increase in 0.25 mg to 0.5 mg increments every 2 weeks as clinically indicated. Divide daily dose to administer for qd or bid dosing. Max dose 6 mg/day in adolescents. | Schizophrenia in adults and adolescents aged 13–17 years<br><br>Alone, or in combination with lithium or valproate, for the short-term treatment of acute manic or mixed episodes associated with Bipolar I Disorder in adults, and alone in children and adolescents aged 10–17 years<br><br>Irritability associated with Autistic Disorder in children and adolescents aged 5–16 years |
| Ziprasidone ⚠️² | Geodon | Tablets: 20, 40, 60, 80 mg<br>IM Injection<br><br>Start at 20 mg daily, increase in 20 mg increments as clinically indicated. Divide daily dose to administer for bid dosing. Max. 160 mg/day in adults. | Schizophrenia in adults<br><br>Acute manic episodes of Bipolar I<br><br>Injection is indicated for the acute treatment of agitation associated with Schizophrenia in adults |

⚠️ ¹ Please see the Black Box Warning "Suicidality and Anitdepressant Drugs" in the Treatment Description section.
⚠️ ² Please see the Black Box Warning "Increased Mortality in Elderly Patients with Dementia-Related Psychosis" in the Treatment Description section.

## Treatment Description:

### FDA Approved Uses:

- Please see Table 1.

### Off-Label Uses:

- Atypical antipsychotics are used for the treatment of psychotic symptoms in youths.
- They are used as monotherapy or as an adjunct for the treatment of manic or mixed symptoms of Bipolar Disorder in youths.
- They can be used for the treatment of agitation in youths.
- They may also be used for the treatment of movement disorders in youths.
- There are off-label uses of this medication and are not FDA approved.

### Black Box Warning

### Suicidality and Antidepressant Drugs

Antidepressants increased the risk compared to placebo of suicidal thinking and behavior (suicidality) in children, adolescents, and young adults in short-term studies of major depressive disorder (MDD) and other psychiatric disorders. Anyone considering the use of any antidepressant in a child, adolescent, or young adult must balance this risk with the clinical need. Short-term studies did not show an increase in the risk of suicidality with antidepressants compared to placebo in adults beyond age 24; there was a reduction in risk with antidepressants compared to placebo in adults aged 65 and older. Depression and certain other psychiatric disorders are themselves associated with increases in the risk of suicide. Patients of all ages who are started on antidepressant therapy should be monitored appropriately and observed closely for clinical worsening, suicidality, or unusual changes in behavior. Families and caregivers should be advised of the need for close observation and communication with the prescriber.

### Black Box Warning

### Increased Mortality in Elderly Patients with Dementia-Related Psychosis

Elderly patients with dementia-related psychosis treated with atypical antipsychotic drugs are at an increased risk of death compared to placebo. Analyses of 17 placebo-controlled trials (modal duration of 10 weeks) in these patients revealed a risk of death in the drug-treated patients of between 1.6 to 1.7 times that seen in placebo-treated patients. Over the course of a typical 10-week controlled trial, the rate of death in drug-treated patients was about 4.5%, compared to a rate of about 2.6% in the placebo group. Although the causes of death were varied, most of the deaths appeared to be either cardiovascular (e.g., heart failure, sudden death) or infectious (e.g., pneumonia) in nature.

### Dosage Forms:

- Please see Table 1.

### Dosing on Initiation:

- Please see Table 1.

### Dosing on Discontinuation:

- Atypical antipsychotic medications should be gradually tapered to avoid any withdrawal side effects.

### Side Effects:

- Sedation, dizziness, as well as anticholinergic side effects such as dry mouth and constipation.
- Extrapyramidal symptoms, increased prolactin, increased QTc interval, and tardive dyskinesia.
- One of the most concerning side effects associated with the use of the atypical antipsychotics is weight gain and metabolic syndrome, with the development of insulin resistance and Type II diabetes.
  - Monitor waist circumference or body mass index, fasting triglyceride levels, fasting HDL cholesterol, fasting glucose, and blood pressure.
- Monitor patients for abnormal involuntary movements (see Figure 1) and extrapyramidal side effects (see Figure 2). Monitor for symptoms of akathesia using the Barnes Akathesia Scale.
- Please check the prescribing information for the medication that you are considering for specific side effect details.

### Contraindications:

- Known hypersensitivity to the medication.
- Use cautiously in patients with hepatic or renal impairment.

### Drug-Drug Interactions:

- Metabolism of certain atypical antipsychotics may be affected by certain medications, such as antidepressants like fluoxetine or paroxetine.
- Avoid certain herbal remedies (valerian, St. John's wort) or agents which may cause sedation or CNS depression as their effects will be additive to those of the atypical antipsychotic.
- Oral contraceptives can potentiate hyperprolactinemia.
- Usage with metoclopramide may increase risk of extrapyramidal symptoms.

## Clinical Pearls

- Risperidone and aripiprazole are the only atypical antipsychotics FDA approved for use in children and adolescents.
- The authors do not recommend long-term management of patients with atypical antipsychotic medications without consultation of a child and adolescent psychiatrist.
- If treating children/adolescents on the autism spectrum, start with a very low dose and be aware of paradoxical or exaggerated responses to medication.

**Figure 1:** Abnormal Involuntary Movement Scale (AIMS)

---

**Exam Procedure:**

Observe the patient at rest before starting the exam. Then, have the patient sit in a hard, firm chair without arm rests. Ask the patient to remove shoes and socks.

- Ask the patient whether there is anything in their mouth and to remove it. Ask about the current condition of teeth, particularly whether dentures are used. (Although not formally a part of the original AIMS, consider whether braces or retainers are in the mouth and whether that is affecting observed oral movements).
  - Are the teeth, dentures, retainers, or braces bothering the patient now?
  - Ask whether any movements in mouth, face, hands, or feet have been noticed. If an affirmative response, obtain description and extent that they bother patient or interfere with activities.
- Ask the patient to sit in a chair with both hands on knees, legs slightly apart, and feet flat on the floor.
  - Observe for any body movements in this position.
- Ask the patient to sit in this position with arms hanging unsupported.
  - Observe for any hand or body movements in this position.
- Ask the patient to open mouth.
  - Observe the tongue for movements at rest within mouth. Repeat once more.
- Ask the patient to protrude tongue.
  - Observe for abnormalities of tongue movement. Repeat once more.
- Ask the patient to tap thumb with each finger as rapidly as possible for 10–15 seconds. Be sure to check for both hands separately.
  - Observe for facial and leg movements.
- Flex and extend patient's arms one at a time.
  - Observe for any rigidity.
- Ask the patient to stand up.
  - Observe the patient in profile and observe all body areas again.
- Ask the patient to extend both arms outstretched in front with palms down.
  - Observe for any trunk, leg, or mouth movements.
- Ask the patient to walk a few paces, turn, and walk back to the chair.
  - Observe hands and gait. Repeat once more.

**Scoring Procedure:**

**Coding:**

1 None – 2 Minimal – 3 Mild – 4 Moderate – 5 Severe

*Facial and Oral Movements:*

1. Muscles of facial expression (e.g., movement of forehead, eyebrows, periorbital area, cheeks; include frowning, blinking, smiling, grimacing)
   1       2       3       4       5

**Figure 1:** Continued

2.  Lips and Perioral Area (e.g., puckering, pouting, smacking)
              1           2           3           4           5

3.  Jaws (e.g., biting, clenching, chewing, mouth opening, lateral movement)
              1           2           3           4           5

4.  Tongue (rate only increase in movement both in and out of mouth, NOT inability to sustain movement.)
              1           2           3           4           5

*Extremity Movements:*

5.  Upper (arms, wrists, hands, fingers). Include choreic movements (e.g., rapid, objectively purposeless, irregular, spontaneous), athetoid movements (e.g., slow, irregular, complex, serpentine). Do NOT include tremor (e.g., repetitive, regular, rhythmic).
              1           2           3           4           5

6.  Lower (legs, knees, ankles, toes) (e.g., lateral knee movement, foot taping, heel dropping, foot squirming, inversion and eversion of foot.)
              1           2           3           4           5

*Trunk Movements:*

7.  Neck, shoulders, hips (e.g., rocking, twisting, squirming, pelvic gyrations)
              1           2           3           4           5

*Global Judgments:*

8.  Severity of abnormal movements:
              1           2           3           4           5

9.  Incapacitation due to abnormal movements:
              1           2           3           4           5

10. Patient's awareness of abnormal movements (rate only patient's report):
              1           2           3           4           5

*Dental Status:*

Current problems with teeth and/or dentures?
              No                    Yes

Does patient usually wear dentures? (Although not formally a part of the AIMS, consider role of braces or retainers.)
              No                    Yes

Adapted from: Department of Health and Human Services; Public Health Service; Alcohol, Drug Abuse, and Mental Health Administration; NIMH Treatment Strategies in Schizophrenia Study, ADM-117; Revised November 1985.

**Figure 2:** Simpson Angus Scale for Extrapyramidal Side Effects

**1. Gait:** Examine patient walking – observe gait, swing of the arms, and general posture.
- 0    Normal
- 1    Diminution of arm swing while walking
- 2    Diminution of arm swing with arm rigidity in the arm
- 3    Stiff gait and arms held rigidly before the abdomen
- 4    Stopped shuffling gait with propulsion and retropulsion

**2. Arm dropping:** Have the patient and the examiner raise both their arms to shoulder height and let them fall to their sides. Normally, a loud slap is heard as the arms hit the sides. Patients with extreme parkinsonian symptoms will have a slow arm drop.
- 0    Normal fall with loud slap and rebound
- 1    Fall slowed slightly with less audible contact and little rebound
- 2    Fall slowed and no rebound
- 3    Marked slowing and no slap
- 4    Arms fall against resistance (as if through glue)

**3. Shoulder shaking:** Have the patient's arms bent at a right angle at the elbow and take one at a time by the examiner. Grasp one hand and also clasp the other around the patient's elbow. The patient's upper arm is pushed back and forth and the humerus is externally rotated. Rate the degree of resistance.
- 0    Normal
- 1    Slight stiffness and resistance
- 2    Moderate stiffness and resistance
- 3    Marked rigidity and difficulty in passive movement
- 4    Extreme stiffness and rigidity with an almost frozen shoulder

**4. Elbow rigidity:** Separately bend the elbow joints at right angles and passively extend and flex them. Observe and palpate the patients biceps. Rate the degree of resistance.
- 0    Normal
- 1    Slight stiffness and resistance
- 2    Moderate stiffness and resistance
- 3    Marked rigidity and difficulty in passive movement
- 4    Extreme stiffness and rigidity with an almost frozen shoulder

**5. Wrist rigidity:** Hold The wrist in one hand and the fingers in the other hand. Extend and flex with ulnar and radial deviation.
- 0    Normal
- 1    Slight stiffness and resistance
- 2    Moderate stiffness and resistance
- 3    Marked rigidity and difficulty in passive movement
- 4    Extreme stiffness and rigidity with an almost frozen shoulder

**Figure 2:** Continued

---

**6. Leg pendulousness:** Have the patient sit on a table with legs hanging down and swinging free. Grasp the ankle and raise it until the knee is partially extended. Allow it to fall and observe the resistance to falling.

  0   The legs swing freely
  1   Slight diminution in the swing of the legs
  2   Moderate resistance to swing
  3   Marked resistance and damping of swing
  4   Complete absence of swing

**7. Head dropping:** Have the patient lie on a well-padded examining table and raise the head with your hand. Withdraw your hand and allow the head to drop. In the normal subject, the head will fall on the table. This movement is delayed in patients with extrapyramidal side effects.

  0   Head falls completely
  1   Slight slowing in fall
  2   Moderate slowing in fall noticeable to the eye
  3   Head falls stiffly and slowly
  4   Head does not reach the examining table

**8. Glabella tap:** Have the patient open the eyes wide and not blink. Tap the glabella region in a steady, rapid speed. Note the number of times the patient blinks in succession.

  0   0–5 blinks
  1   6–10 blinks
  2   11–15 blinks
  3   16–20 blinks
  4   21 and more blinks

**9. Tremor:** Observe the patient walking into examining room and then reexamine:

  0   Normal
  1   Mild finger tremor
  2   Tremor of the hand or arm occurring spasmodically
  3   Persistent tremor of one or more limbs
  4   Whole body tremor

**10. Salivation**: Observe the patient while talking. Ask the patient to open the mouth and elevate the tongue.

  0   Normal
  1   Excess salivation with pooling of saliva.
  2   Excess salivation with occasional difficulty in speaking
  3   Difficulty speaking due to excess salivation
  4   Frank drooling

Adapted from Simpson GM, Angus JWS. A rating scale for extrapyramidal side effects. Acta Psychiatr Scand. 1970;212:11-19.

---

# 26 Benzodiazepines

**Medications Discussed in this Chapter:**

- Alprazolam
- Lorazepam
- Clonazepam

There are many agents that fall under the category of benzodiazepines. In narrowing the list of medications to those that are effective and provide a clinically distinctive response, short-acting preparations of alprazolam, lorazepam, and clonazepam stand out (see Table 1 for a comparison of these agents).

There are few classes of medication in psychiatry, outside of the psychostimulants, which can alleviate symptoms as rapidly. For certain indications, such as severe anxiety symptoms that require more immediate treatment than waiting four to six weeks for an SSRI to take effect, benzodiazepines can fill a needed void in the pharmacological portion of the treatment plan.

It is important to note that benzodiazepines should be short-term interventions meant to serve as a stop gap until symptoms are under better control. Due to the risk of dependence, as well as the potential for paradoxical reactions in some children and adolescents, they should be used judiciously and tapered off as soon as clinically possible.

**Table 1:**

| Generic Name | Brand Name | Dosages (mg) | Side Effects | Monitoring |
|---|---|---|---|---|
| Alprazolam | Xanax | Tablets: 0.25, 0.5, 1, 2 mg<br><br>Oral Solution:<br><br>0.25, 0.5, 1/5ml, 0.25/2.5ml<br><br>Initial dose of 0.005 mg/kg/dose or 0.125 mg/dose tid | Sedation, disinhibition, incoordination, confusion, memory impairment | Heart rate and pulse, blood pressure, CBC, liver function |

**Table 1:** Continued

| Generic Name | Brand Name | Dosages (mg) | Side Effects | Monitoring |
|---|---|---|---|---|
| | | Increase in increments of 0.125–0.25 mg up to a maximum of 0.02 mg/kg/dose or 0.06 mg/kg/day | | |
| | | (0.375–3mg/day) | | |
| Lorazepam | Ativan | Tablets: 0.5, 1, 2 mg<br><br>Oral solution: 2 mg/ml<br><br>IM: 2/ml, 4/ml<br><br>0.02–0.1mg/kg every 4–8 hours | Sedation, disinhibition, incoordination, confusion, memory impairment | Heart rate and pulse, blood pressure, CBC |
| Clonazapam | Klonopin | Tablets: 0.5, 1, 2 mg<br><br>0.1–0.2 mg/kg/day in two divided doses | Sedation, disinhibition, incoordination, confusion, memory impairment | Heart rate and pulse, blood pressure, CBC, liver function |

# Benzodiazepine Medications

## Treatment Description

### FDA Approved Uses:

- Management of anxiety disorders or short-term relief of symptoms of anxiety.
- Treatment of panic disorder, with or without agoraphobia.
- Treatment of seizures, including status epilepticus for lorazepam.
- Alprazolam is approved for use in patients above 18 years of age, lorazepam in patients above 12 years of age, and clonazepam in patients above 18 years of age.

### Off-Label Uses:

- Benzodiazepines can be useful interventions for short-term treatment of moderate to severe anxiety disorders. They can be used to relieve anxiety symptoms until a selective serotonin reuptake inhibitor (SSRI) has become therapeutic.

- They may also be used for the short-term treatment of sleep disorders. This should not be done without a proper trial of behavioral interventions including sleep hygiene. Refer to Appendix E for additional information.
- They can be used for the treatment of alcohol withdrawal.

## Black Box Warnings:

- None

## Dosage Forms:

- Please refer to Table 1.
- 

## Dosing on Initiation:

- Please refer to Table 1

## Dosing on Discontinuation:

- Benzodiazepines should be gradually tapered to avoid any withdrawal side effects or rebound anxiety. Slowly decreasing the dose every three to four days should be well tolerated (may need to taper more slowly if using longer-acting benzodiazepine.)

## Side Effects:

- Side effects of benzodiazepines include sedation, irritability, behavioral disinhibition, and cognitive impairment.
- Decreased respiratory drive, confusion, and coma can occur at higher doses.
- Due to the risk of dependence, benzodiazepines should be used only briefly.

## Contraindications:

- Known hypersensitivity to the medication.
- Acute narrow angle glaucoma.
- Use cautiously in patients with substance abuse issues.

## Drug-Drug Interactions:

- Use of valerian, kava kava, St. John's wort, narcotics, barbiturates, or cimetidine (Tagamet) should be avoided as CNS depression can be increased.
- Oral contraceptives may decrease the clearance of benzodiazepines.

## Clinical Pearls

- Many benzodiazepines are available including newer extended release preparations. As with most medications, use caution in prescribing newer agents to children and adolescents, particularly when being used off-label.

- Only three agents are listed in this chapter to simplify selection of an appropriate agent. By choosing among these three agents, you will be able to treat most patients. The major difference between the agents is time of onset and duration of effect.

  - Onset of action from fastest to slowest is alprazolam, lorazepam, and clonazepam. Duration of effect from longest to shortest is clonazepam, lorazepam, and then alprazolam.

  - A time course of symptoms through the day may be helpful in determining which agent to select. For example, patients with symptoms throughout the day may do better with tid dosing of clonazepam. However, the child with acute onset of anxiety symptoms at random short-lived times of the day may do better with alprazolam.

  - For patients with anxiety, you can prescribe less benzodiazepines with effective standing doses than to catch up with prn doses once the anxiety has set in.

- Paradoxical reactions to benzodiazepines can occur. Watch for increased irritability, restlessness, agitation, aggression, hallucinations, and nightmares.

- The disadvantages of these medications are sedation, potential for disinhibition, physical and psychological dependence. Therefore, their use in children and adolescents should be used not as maintenance medications, but as an aid in the acute management of severe anxiety (i.e., severe school avoidance) for a brief period. Avoid long-term use of benzodiazepines due to the risk of dependence.

# 27 Mood Stabilizers

## Medications Discussed in this Chapter:

- Lithium
- Valproate*

There are many agents that fall under the category of mood stabilizers. In narrowing the list of medications to those that are effective and have a known, manageable side effect profile, lithium and valproate stand out (see Table 1 for a comparison of these agents). The diagnosis and treatment of bipolar disorder is, in our professional opinion, reaching the edges of what can be safely and effectively managed by the pediatrician or PCP without consultation of a specialist. This information is provided for those who feel comfortable with prescribing and managing mood stabilizers.

As this list may seem too narrow to some, we also include a short synopsis of our rational. A key point to keep in mind is that for patients with bipolar disorder, there is much controversy about the diagnosis to begin with and how broadly to define the phenotype of symptoms.

There are inherent difficulties with obtaining blood levels and some level of greater follow-up is required with these two agents. However, if bipolar disorder is diagnosed in the primary care setting, one could also argue that careful and thorough follow-up to continue the assessment process (and further confirm the diagnosis) as well as to ensure a safe and efficacious medication trial is advantageous. According to the AACAP Practice Parameters, atypical antipsychotic medications may also be considered. We would urge caution due to the significant side effects of these medications (see Chapter 25), such as metabolic syndrome and Stevens-Johnson syndrome. Serious consideration should be given for a specialist consultation with a child and adolescent psychiatrist to verify the diagnosis as well as to provide on-going care and expertise for medication trials and treatment.

Also, there is a tendency for polypharmacy in the treatment of bipolar disorder. Our hope is that before a child is started on multiple medications that a consultation with a child and adolescent psychiatrist is considered. In the case that a patient has significantly acute symptoms requiring treatment with a mood stabilizer in combination with an antipsychotic medication, we would recommend that the patient receive a consultation with a child and adolescent psychiatrist before routine management occurs with a pediatrician or PCP.

Lastly, as much as there are anecdotal accounts for the efficacy of many medications (for example, gabapentin), later systematic trials have revealed that initial hype does not necessarily translate to efficacy and tolerability. Particularly if bipolar disorder is to be diagnosed and treated in the primary care setting, we suggest the use of agents that have an evidence base, so that, if a child does not improve, there

---

* When referring to the term "valproate" in this chapter, we are referring to all forms of this medication including valproic acid, divalproex sodium, and valproate sodium. We do not differentiate between the specific forms to simplify the presentation of the material. Please refer to the prescribing information for each medication for additional information prior to prescribing.

is less of a question whether the problem was in selecting the wrong medication or in having the wrong diagnosis to begin with.

To reiterate, in our professional opinion, the diagnosis and treatment of bipolar disorder requires diagnostic skill and pharmacological expertise. Consultation with a child and adolescent psychiatrist should be considered for its assessment and treatment. Patients who are stable and are on an appropriate medication regimen may be managed by a pediatrician or PCP.

**Table 1:**    Comparison of Lithium and Valproate

| Generic Name | Brand Name | Dosages (mg) | Side Effects | Monitoring |
|---|---|---|---|---|
| Lithium Carbonate △ 1 | Lithobid (SR), Eskalith (CR) | Capsules: 150, 300, 600 mg Syrup: 300 mg/5ml Tablets: 300 mg Tablet, controlled release (Eskalith CR): 450 mg Tablet, slow release (Lithobid): 300 mg<br><br>Children: 15–60 mg/kg/day in 3–4 divided doses<br><br>Adolescents: 600–1800 mg/day in 3–4 divided doses or 2 divided doses for sustained release | Sedation, thirst, polyuria, polydipsia, visual changes, tremor, hypothyroidism, acne | Thyroid function tests, plasma concentrations. Serum levels: 0.6–1.2 mEq/L |
| Valproate △ 2 | Depakote, Depakene, Depacon | Capsule (Depakene): 250 mg Capsule, sprinkles (Depakote sprinkles): 125 mg Syrup: 250 mg/5 ml Tablets, delayed release (Depakote): 125, 250, 500 mg Tablet, extended release (Depakote ER): 250, 500 mg<br><br>Injection (Depacon): 10–15 mg/kg/day IV divided up to tid, max 60 mg/kg/day | Sedation, thrombocytopenia, alopecia, tremor, hepatotozicity, agranulocytosis, neutropenia | CBC with platelets, liver function tests, plasma concentrations: Serum level: 50–125 micrograms/ml |

 [1]    Please see the Black Box Warning in the Lithium part of the Treatment Description section.

△ [2]    Please see the Black Box Warning in the Valproate part of the Treatment Description section.

## Lithium (Eskalith, Eskalith CR, Lithobid, Lithobid SR):

### Treatment Description

#### FDA Approved Uses:

- Treatment of manic episodes of bipolar disorder.
- Maintenance treatment for individuals with a diagnosis of bipolar disorder.
- It is approved for adolescents 12 years and older.

#### Off-Label Uses:

- Lithium is used off-label for the treatment of the above listed indications in children younger than 12 years of age.
- Lithium is also used as an augmentation agent for the treatment of depression. It is also used for migraine and cluster headaches. There are off-label uses of this medication and are not FDA approved.

 **Black Box Warning**

Lithium toxicity is closely related to serum lithium levels, and can occur at doses close to therapeutic levels. Facilities for prompt and accurate serum lithium determinations should be available before initiating therapy.

#### Dosage Forms:

- Please refer to Table 1.

#### Dosing on Initiation:

- Immediate-release capsules should be given three to four times a day while extended release tablets should be given twice daily (at approximately 12-hour intervals).
- Dosing should be guided by steady state serum levels and clinical response.
- Start with a test dose to assess for tolerability. Gradually increase the dose based upon serial serum levels and clinical response.
- Rapid dosage escalations are associated with greater side effects such as nausea, diarrhea, hand tremor, and urinary frequency. Gradual increases, particularly in the outpatient setting, are suggested.
- Target lithium level should be between 0.6 and 1.2 mEq/L. Please note that there is a narrow therapeutic range beyond which toxic levels can be quickly reached.

#### Dosing on Discontinuation:

- Lithium should be gradually tapered to avoid any withdrawal side effects.

## Side Effects:

- Fine tremor, increased thirst, and polyuria.

- Nausea, diarrhea, vomiting, weight gain, drowsiness, muscular weakness, and lack of coordination may also occur.

- Ataxia, giddiness, tinnitus, blurred vision, and a large output of dilute urine may be seen with high or near toxic levels.

- Abnormalities in renal function and changes in morphologic structure can occur.

- Impaired thyroid function including hypothyroidism, euthyroid goiter, and hyperthyroidism are possible.

## Contraindications:

- Known hypersensitivity to the medication.

- Use cautiously in patients with renal impairment, cardiovascular disease, significant thyroid disease, dehydration or sodium depletion.

- Avoid in pregnant women, particularly early in pregnancy.

## Drug-Drug Interactions:

- Caffeine may lower lithium serum concentrations.

- Nonsteroidal anti-inflammatory drugs and other drugs which alter sodium excretion may lead to increased lithium serum concentrations.

- The risk for neurotoxicity of lithium may be increased if combined with SSRI medications or carbamazepine.

- Lithium levels should be closely monitored when patients initiate or discontinue nonsteroidal anti-inflammatory drugs (NSAIDs) due to risk of lithium toxicity.

## Clinical Pearls

- Adverse reactions may be encountered with serum lithium levels below 1.5 mEq/L. Mild to moderate adverse reactions may occur at levels from 1.5 to 2.5 mEq/L, and moderate to severe reactions may be seen at levels of 2.0 mEq/L and above.

- It is important to explain, preferably with written instructions, about obtaining lithium levels for patients and families. It is important that they understand that you want a trough level, i.e., that you need to measure the lowest level of lithium in their body before their next scheduled dose.

- As side effects may increase with rapid dose titrations, it is advisable to adjust the dose of lithium on a weekly basis. It is important that patients and parents understand the potential side effects of lithium as well as signs of potential lithium toxicity.

- Due to the potential for significant toxicity in overdose, it is recommended that parents store and administer the medication to the patient.

## Valproate (Depakote, Depakene)

### Treatment Description

#### FDA Approved Uses:

- Treatment of multiple seizure types.
    - Use with extreme caution under age 2 years due to risk for fatal hepatotoxicity.
- Treatment of manic episodes of bipolar disorder.
    - Not approved for patients under age 18 for treatment of manic episodes.
    - FDA approved for divalproex sodium only.
- Prophylaxis of migraine headaches
    - Not approved for patients under age 16 years for prophylaxis of migraine headaches.
    - FDA approved for divalproex sodium only.

#### Off-Label Uses:

- Valproate is used off label for the treatment of bipolar disorder in youths younger than 18 years of age.
- This is an off-label use of this medication and is not FDA approved.

 **Black Box Warnings**

### Hepatoxicity:

Hepatic failure resulting in fatalities has occurred in patients receiving valproic acid and its derivatives. Experience has indicated that children under the age of two years are at a considerably increased risk of developing fatal hepatotoxicity, especially those on multiple anticonvulsants, those with congenital metabolic disorders, those with severe seizure disorders accompanied by mental retardation, and those with organic brain disease. When Depakote is used in this patient group, it should be used with extreme caution as a sole agent. The benefits of therapy should be weighed against the risks. Above this age group, experience in epilepsy has indicated that the incidence of fatal hepatotoxicity decreases considerably in progressively older patient groups. These incidents usually have occurred during the first six months of treatment. Serious or fatal hepatotoxicity may be preceded by nonspecific symptoms malaise, weakness, lethargy, facial edema, anorexia, and vomiting. In patients with epilepsy, a loss of seizure control may also occur. Patients should be monitored closely for the appearance of these symptoms. Liver function tests should be performed prior to therapy and at frequent intervals thereafter, especially during the first six months.

### Teratogenicity:

Valproate can produce teratogenic effects such as neural tube defects (e.g., spina bifida). Accordingly, the use of depakote tablets in women of childbearing potential requires that the benefits of its use be weighed against the risk of injury to the fetus. This is especially important when the treatment of a spontaneously reversible condition not ordinarily associated with permanent injury or risk of death (e.g., migraine) is contemplated.

## Pancreatitis:

Cases of life-threatening pancreatitis have been reported in both children and adults receiving valproate. Some of the cases have been described as hemorrhagic with a rapid progression from initial symptoms to death. Cases have been reported shortly after initial use as well as after several years of use. Patients and guardians should be warned that abdominal pain, nausea, vomiting, and/or anorexia can be symptoms of pancreatitis that require prompt medical evaluation. If pancreatitis is diagnosed, valproate should ordinarily be discontinued. Alternative treatment for the underlying medical condition should be initiated as clinically indicated.

### Dosage Forms:

- Please refer to Table 1.

### Dosing on Initiation:

- Immediate-release capsules should be given three to four times a day while extended release tablets should be given twice daily (at approximately 12-hour intervals).
- Dosing should be guided by steady state serum levels and clinical response.
- Start with a test dose to assess for tolerability. Gradually increase the dose based upon serial serum levels and clinical response.
- Rapid dosage escalations are associated with greater side effects such as nausea, diarrhea, hand tremor, and urinary frequency. Gradual increases, particularly in the outpatient setting, are suggested.
- Target valproate level should be between 50 and 125 ug/ml.

### Dosing on Discontinuation:

- Valproate should be gradually tapered to avoid any withdrawal side effects.

### Side Effects:

- Nausea, vomiting, dizziness, somnolence, asthenia, and dyspepsia may occur.
- Increased appetite, weight gain, diplopia, blurry vision, and alopecia have also been reported.
- Hyperammonemia can occur. In particular, patients with urea cycle disorders may suffer hyperammonemic encephalopathy and death.
- Thrombocytopenia, multi-organ hypersensitivity reaction, and polycystic ovary syndrome are possible.
- Please refer to black box warning above for additional side effects.

### Contraindications:

- Known hypersensitivity to the medication
- Patients with hepatic disease or significant hepatic dysfunction.
- Use cautiously in pregnant women due to risk of teratogenicity.

### Drug-Drug Interactions:

- Use caution in using medications which would affect the clearance of valproate and/or other coadministered medications. For example, phenytoin or carbamazepine may double the clearance of valproate. Likewise, valproate can increase the elimination half-life of lamictal from 26 to 70 hours thus increasing risk of Stevens-Johnson syndrome and toxic epidermal necrolysis.
- Combining valproate with salicylates may lead to acute toxicity.
- Serum concentrations of valproic acid may be decreased if taken with food.
- Valproate may increase the central nervous system depressant effects of other medications.

### Clinical Pearls

- It is important to explain, preferably with written instructions, about obtaining valproate levels for patients and families. It is important that they understand that you want a trough level, i.e., that you need to measure the lowest level of valproate in their body before their next scheduled dose.
- As side effects may increase with rapid dose titrations, it is advisable to adjust the dose of valproate on a weekly basis. It is important that patients and parents understand the potential side effects of valproate as well as signs of potential valproate toxicity.
- It is recommended that parents store and administer the medication to the patient.

# 28 Stimulants and Related ADHD Medications

## Medications Discussed in this Chapter:

- Stimulant Medications
  - Amphetamine Preparations
    - Adderall
    - Adderall XR
    - Dexedrine
    - Dexedrine Spansule
    - DextroStat
    - Lisdexamfetamine
  - Methylphenidate Preparations
    - Concerta
    - Daytrana Patch
    - Focalin
    - Focalin XR
    - Metadate CD
    - Metadate ER
    - Methylin
    - Methylin ER
    - Ritalin
    - Ritalin SR
- Nonstimulant ADHD medications
  - Atomoxetine
  - Bupropion (see Chapter 24: Antidepressants)
  - Clonidine (See Chapter 23: Alpha Adrenergic Agonists)
  - Guanfacine (See Chapter 23: Alpha Adrenergic Agonists)

Stimulant medications are the first line of treatment for ADHD. There is no strong evidence to indicate improved efficacy between methylphenidate preparations and amphetamine preparations. Selection of stimulant medication is based more so on time course of symptoms throughout the day, the individual patient's response to a particular medication, and the tolerability of that medication for a particular patient.

Stimulants are also used to a much lesser extent as augmentation agents in the treatment of depression in specific clinical situations. This is an off-label use. It is suggested that patients unresponsive to monotherapy for the treatment of depression be referred for specialist care by a child and adolescent psychiatrist.

Nonstimulant medications for the treatment of ADHD symptoms include atomoxetine, bupropion, clonidine, and guanfacine. The authors of this text recommend using stimulants as the first line treatment of choice for the management of ADHD. Atomoxetine is FDA approved for ADHD and may be considered a first line treatment, however, the authors suggest that pediatricians and PCPs use stimulants as the preferred first line treatment. The main concern arises, in our professional opinion, when balancing the relative efficacy of atomoxetine with the potential for significant effects on mood and its black box warning regarding suicidal ideation. This is of greater concern in the primary care setting where certain practice realities, such as the lack of time for comprehensive psychiatric evaluation and variability of expertise across providers, may create a greater potential to miss an underlying or comorbid mood disorder.

There are also older tricyclic antidepressants and monoamine oxidase inhibitors which can be used for the management of ADHD, such as imipramine and nortriptyline. It is suggested that patients unresponsive to the stimulant and nonstimulant medications discussed in this chapter be referred for specialist care by a child and adolescent psychiatrist.

Please note that this chapter presents information on multiple different medications. For the ease of presenting a large amount of data, multiple pieces of information have been incorporated. In certain cases, if a side effect or contraindication is common to multiple medications, but not all, it has been listed below so that providers are aware of the potential of such a side effect. Before selecting any specific medication, please be sure to reference the current prescribing information from the manufacturer for that specific drug for additional information.

## Stimulant Medications

### Treatment Description

#### FDA Approved Uses:

- Stimulants are FDA approved for the treatment of ADHD and narcolepsy. Dextroamphetamine is also approved for the treatment of exogenous obesity. All methylphenidate preparations are approved in children 6 years of age or older. Most amphetamine preparations are approved in children 3 years of age or older.

#### Off-Label Uses:

- Stimulants are also used as augmentation agents for the treatment of depression. This is an off-label use of these medications and is not FDA approved.

**Black Box Warnings**

- Amphetamines have a high potential for abuse. Administration of amphetamines for prolonged periods of time may lead to drug dependence. Particular attention should be paid to the possibility of patients obtaining prescribed amphetamines for nontherapeutic use or distribution of the drug to others. The drugs should be prescribed or dispensed sparingly.

- Misuse of amphetamine may cause sudden death and serious cardiovascular adverse events.

### Dosage Forms:

- Please refer to Table 1.

### Dosing on Initiation:

- Please refer to Table 1.

### Dosing on Discontinuation:

- Stimulants may be discontinued quickly if clinically indicated. However, a gradual taper may be better tolerated and may decrease the likelihood of a rebound in ADHD symptoms.

**Table 1:**   Review of Current Stimulant Medications

| Generic Name | Brand Name | Dosages (mg) | Typical Start-ing Dose | FDA Max/Day | Off-Label Max/Day |
|---|---|---|---|---|---|
| Amphetamine preparation – short-acting ⚠ | Adderall | Tablets: 5, 7.5, 10, 12.5, 15, 20, 30 mg | 3–5 years: 2.5 mg qd > 6 years: 5 mg qd-bid | 40 mg | > 50 kg: 60 mg |
| Amphetamine preparation – short-acting ⚠ | Dexedrine | Tablets: 5, 10 mg | 3–5 years: 2.5 mg qd > 6 y: 5 mg qd-bid | | |
| Amphetamine preparation – short-acting ⚠ | DextroStat | Capsules: 5, 10 mg | > 6 years: 5 mg qd-bid | | |

**Table 1:** Continued

| Generic Name | Brand Name | Dosages (mg) | Typical Starting Dose | FDA Max/Day | Off-Label Max/Day |
|---|---|---|---|---|---|
| Amphetamine preparation – long-acting ⚠ | Dexedrine Spansule | Capsules: 5, 10, 15mg | >6 years: 5–10 mg qd-bid | 40 mg | > 50 kg: 60 mg |
| Amphetamine preparation – long-acting ⚠ | Adderall XR | Capsules: 5, 10, 15, 20, 25, 30 mg | >6 y: 10 mg qd | 70 mg | Not yet known |
| Amphetamine preparation – long-acting ⚠ | Lisdexamfetamine | Capsules: 30, 50, 70 mg | 30 mg qd | 70 mg | Not yet known |
| Methylphenidate preparation – short-acting ⚠ | Focalin | Capsules: 2.5, 5, 10 mg | 2.5 mg bid | 20 mg | 50 mg |
| Methylphenidate preparation – short-acting ⚠ | Methylin | Tablets: 5, 10, 20 mg | 5 mg bid | 60 mg | > 50 kg: 100 mg |
| Methylphenidate preparation – short acting ⚠ | Ritalin | Tablets: 5, 10, 20 mg | 5 mg bid | 60 mg | > 50 kg: 100 mg |
| Methylphenidate preparation – intermediate-acting ⚠ | Metadate ER | Capsules: 10, 20 mg | 10 mg qam | 60 mg | > 50 kg: 100 mg |
| Methylphenidate preparation – intermediate-acting ⚠ | Ritalin SR | Tablet: 20 mg | 10 mg qam | 60 mg | > 50 kg: 100 mg |

**Table 1:** Continued

| Generic Name | Brand Name | Dosages (mg) | Typical Starting Dose | FDA Max/Day | Off-Label Max/Day |
|---|---|---|---|---|---|
| Methylphenidate preparation – intermediate-acting ⚠ | Metadate CD | Tablets: 10, 20, 30, 40, 50, 60 mg | 20 mg qam | 60 mg | > 50 kg: 100 mg |
| Methylphenidate preparation – intermediate-acting ⚠ | Methylin oral and Methylin chewables | Oral solution: 5mg/5ml, 10 mg/5mg Chewable tablets: 2.5, 5, 10 mg | 10 mg qam | 60 mg | > 50 mg: 100 mg |
| Methylphenidate preparation – long-acting ⚠ | Concerta | Caplets: 18, 27, 36, 54 mg | 18 mg qam | 72 mg | 108 mg |
| Methylphenidate preparation – long-acting ⚠ | Focalin XR | Capsules: 5, 10, 15, 20 mg | 5 mg qam | 30 mg | 50 mg |
| Methylphenidate preparation – long-acting ⚠ | Daytrana patch | Patches: 10, 15, 20, 30 mg | Begin with 10 mg patch qd, titrate up by patch strength 5 mg qam | 30 mg | Not yet known |

⚠ Please see the previous section: Black Box Warnings.

## Side Effects:

- The most common side effects are decreased appetite, GI upset, weight loss, and insomnia. Weight and height should be monitored serially to ensure appropriate growth and development.

- Stimulants may increase blood pressure and heart rate. Serious cardiovascular events, including sudden death, have been reported in patients with preexisting structural cardiac abnormalities and other serious heart conditions.

  - There was a recent recommendation from the American Heart Association for routine electrocardiograms in all youths being considered for a trial of stimulant medication. This statement was later modified. Due to the recent nature of this announcement, the press release reviewing the recommendations at the time of publication of this text is provided in Figure 1. As this is a topic that may further develop, readers are advised to verify current recommendations when considering the prescribing of stimulant medications.

- Stimulants may affect psychiatric symptoms as well.
  - They may worsen preexisting psychosis or lead to treatment emergent psychotic symptoms.
  - They may increase risk of mania or mixed mood episodes in patients with bipolar disorder. They may also lead to treatment emergent manic symptoms.
  - There may be depressive symptoms or a worsening of depressed mood.
  - There may be an increase in aggression for some patients.
  - They may worsen tics and OCD symptoms.
- There may be long-term suppression of growth, an increase in risk of seizure, as well as development of difficulties with vision, such as in accommodation and blurring of vision.

**Figure 1:** American Academy of Pediatrics and American Heart Association Clarification of Statement on Cardiovascular Evaluation and Monitoring of Children and Adolescents With Heart Disease Receiving Medications for ADHD

The American Heart Association released on April 21, 2008, a statement about cardiovascular evaluation and monitoring of children receiving drugs for the treatment of Attention Deficit Hyperactivity Disorder (ADHD). As a result of language in the news release and the statement as published, there have been conflicting interpretations of the recommendations regarding the use of an electrocardiogram (ECG) in assessing children with ADHD who may need treatment with medications. The purpose of this joint advisory of the American Academy of Pediatrics (AAP) and the American Heart Association (AHA) is to clarify the recommendations. This clarification has been endorsed by the American Academy of Child and Adolescent Psychiatry, the American College of Cardiology, Children and Adults with Attention-Deficit/Hyperactivity Disorder and the National Initiative for Children's Healthcare Quality.

- The scientific statement included a review of data that show children with heart conditions have a higher incidence of ADHD.

- Because certain heart conditions in children may be difficult (even, in some cases, impossible) to detect, the AAP and AHA feel that it is prudent to carefully assess children for heart conditions who need to receive treatment with drugs for ADHD.

- Obtaining a patient and family health history and doing a physical exam focused on cardiovascular disease risk factors (Class I recommendations in the statement) are recommended by the AAP and AHA for assessing patients before treatment with drugs for ADHD.

- Acquiring an ECG is a Class IIa recommendation. This means that it is reasonable for a physician to consider obtaining an ECG as part of the evaluation of children being considered for stimulant drug therapy, but this should be at the physician's judgment, and it is not mandatory to obtain one.

- Treatment of a patient with ADHD should not be withheld because an ECG is not done. The child's physician is the best person to make the assessment about whether there is a need for an ECG.

- Medications that treat ADHD have not been shown to cause heart conditions nor have they been demonstrated to cause sudden cardiac death. However, some of these medications can increase or decrease heart rate and blood pressure. While these side effects are not usually considered dangerous, they should be monitored in children with heart conditions as the physician feels necessary.

An erratum to the statement has been developed to clarify the language and to assure that the intent is clear to all readers. This is available at: http://circ.ahajournals.org/cgi/content/full/CIRCULATIONAHA.107.189473/DC1

**Contraindications:**

- Known hypersensitivity to the medication.

- Patients with marked anxiety, tension, and agitation, since the drug may aggravate these symptoms.

- Patients being treated with monoamine oxidase (MAO) inhibitors, and also within a minimum of 14 days following discontinuation of a MAO-inhibitor (hypertensive crises may result).

- Patients with glaucoma.

- Patients with motor tics or with a family history or diagnosis of Tourette's syndrome.

**Drug-Drug Interactions:**

- Significant interactions are reviewed below. Before selecting any specific medication, please be sure to reference the current prescribing information from the manufacturer for that specific drug for additional information.

- Antihistamines – Stimulants may counteract the sedative effect of antihistamines.

- Lithium – The anorectic and stimulatory effects of stimulants may be inhibited by lithium.

- MAO Inhibitors – Use of stimulants with MAOI antidepressants can cause headaches and other signs of hypertensive crisis. A variety of toxic neurological effects and malignant hyperpyrexia can occur, sometimes with fatal results.

- Phenobarbital and Phenytoin – Stimulants may produce a synergistic anticonvulsant action.

- Tricyclic Antidepressants – Use of stimulants with tricyclic antidepressants may enhance the activity of both substances.

## Clinical Pearls

- Short-acting preparations last 3½ to 4 hours, intermediate-acting preparations last 6–8 hours, and long-acting medications last from 8–12 hours.

- Short-acting stimulants are often used as initial treatment in children but have the disadvantage of bid to tid dosing to control symptoms throughout the day. Long-acting stimulants offer greater convenience and compliance with a single daily dose; however, these may have greater effects on evening appetite and sleep.

- To begin a trial of stimulant, begin with a short acting preparation. In case the patient has any side effects, paradoxical reactions, or untoward effects, the time course of symptoms can be significantly shorter.

- Stimulant trials are one of the few areas of psychopharmacology where immediate results are seen. Titrate dosing as clinically indicated. Switching to a long-acting preparation will improve compliance.

- Adderall XR, Metadate CD, and Ritalin LA capsules may be opened and sprinkled on food.

- Methylin also has chewable and liquid preparations.

- Methylphenidate preparations are not FDA approved for use in children under the age of 6 years.

- In children with mood issues as well as ADHD, treat the mood symptoms first, then the ADHD. One of the common reasons that children with ADHD do not optimally respond to stimulants is that there are undiagnosed mood disorders that have not been stabilized. Likewise, if a patient becomes increasingly moody or irritable, take a step back and consider whether there were mood symptoms that you may have overlooked.

- Consider using a methylphenidate preparation rather than an amphetamine preparation first in a child with a history of anxiety or dysthymia.

- Rebound symptoms in the late afternoon/early evening (i.e., irritability, hyperactivity, or difficulty sleeping) may be improved with the addition of a small dose of short-acting medication in the late afternoon.

## Nonstimulant ADHD medications
*Atomoxetine (Strattera)*

### Treatment Description

#### FDA Approved Uses:

- Atomoxetine is FDA approved for the treatment of ADHD in children, adolescents, and adults.

#### Off-Label Uses:

- Atomoxetine has no other significant off-label uses.

### Black Box Warnings

#### Suicidal Ideation in Children and Adolescents

Strattera (atomoxetine) increased the risk of suicidal ideation in short-term studies in children or adolescents with Attention Deficit Hyperactivity Disorder (ADHD). Anyone considering the use of Strattera in a child or adolescent must balance this risk with clinical need. Patients who are started on therapy should be monitored closely for suicidality (suicidal thinking and behavior), clinical worsening, or unusual changes in behavior. Families and caregivers should be advised of the need for close observation and communication with the prescriber. Strattera is approved for ADHD in pediatric and adult patients. Strattera is not approved for major depressive disorder. Pooled analyses of short-term (6 to 18 weeks) placebo-controlled trials of Strattera in children and adolescents (a total of 12 trials involving over 2200 patients, including 11 trials in ADHD and 1 trial in enuresis) have revealed a greater risk of suicidal ideation early during treatment in those receiving Strattera compared to placebo. The average risk of suicidal ideation in patients receiving Strattera was 0.4% (5/1357 patients), compared to none in placebo-treated patients (851 patients). No suicides occurred in these trials.

All pediatric patients being treated with Strattera should be monitored closely for suicidality, clinical worsening, and unusual changes in behavior, especially during the initial few months of a course of drug therapy, or at times of dose changes. Such monitoring would generally include at least weekly face-to-face contact with patients or their family members or caregivers during the first 4 weeks of treatment, then fortnightly visits for the next 4 weeks, then at 12 weeks, and as clinically indicated beyond 12 weeks. Additional contact by telephone may be appropriate between face-to-face visits.

## Dosage Forms:

- Capsules: 10 mg, 18 mg, 25 mg, 40 mg, 60 mg, 80 mg, and 100 mg

## Dosing on Initiation:

- Optimal dosing is 1.2 mg/kg/d which can be increased to 1.4 mg/kg/d (label use) or 1.8 mg/kg/d (off-label).
- Start slowly: For children and adolescents < 70 kg: start at 0.5 mg/kg for 2 weeks and, if tolerated, increase to 1.2 mg/kg/d.
- Give medication once or twice daily. Typically start in one dose after dinner. You can convert it to once daily dosing in the morning if preferred.
- It takes up to 4–6 weeks to reach maximum therapeutic effect.

## Dosing on Discontinuation:

- A gradual taper may be better tolerated and may decrease potential for withdrawal side effects.

## Side Effects:

- The most common side effects are sedation, stomachaches, headache, nausea, and vomiting. These are helped by dosing it after dinner.
- Effects on blood pressure and pulse were noted and should be monitored during treatment.
- Severe liver injury has been reported. It should be discontinued in patients with jaundice or laboratory evidence of liver injury, and should not be restarted.
- Sudden death has been reported in association with atomoxetine treatment at usual doses in children and adolescents with structural cardiac abnormalities or other serious heart problems.
- Atomoxetine may affect psychiatric symptoms as well.
  - It may worsen preexisting psychosis or lead to treatment emergent psychotic symptoms.
  - It may increase risk of mania or mixed mood episodes in patients with bipolar disorder. It may also lead to treatment emergent manic symptoms.
  - It may increase aggression or hostility for some patients.
  - It may increase risk of urinary retention and urinary hesitation. Rare cases of priapism have also been reported.
  - Some patients have experienced allergic reactions including angioneurotic edema, urticaria, and rash.

### Contraindications:

- Known hypersensitivity to atomoxetine.

- It should not be taken with an MAOI, or within 2 weeks after discontinuing an MAOI. Treatment with an MAOI should not be initiated within 2 weeks after discontinuing atomoxetine. Cases have occurred with features resembling neuroleptic malignant syndrome.

- Presence of narrow angle glaucoma.

### Drug-Drug Interactions:

- Significant interactions are reviewed below. Before selecting any specific medication, please be sure to reference the current prescribing information from the manufacturer for that specific drug for additional information.

- *Albuterol* – Use of atomoxetine in combination with albuterol should be done cautiously due to the potential for increased heart rate and blood pressure.

- *CYP2D6 Inhibitors* – Use of atomoxetine with inhibitors of CYP2D6 (i.e., quinidine, fluoxetine, and paroxetine) can increase atomoxetine plasma levels, as well as half-life, due to decreased metabolism in extensive metabolizers.

- *MAO Inhibitors* – Use of atomoxetine with MAOI antidepressants can precipitate symptoms resembling neuroleptic malignant syndrome.

- *Pressor Agents* – It should be used cautiously with pressor agents (i.e., dopamine or dobutamine) due to effects on blood pressure.

- *Tricyclic Antidepressants* – Use of stimulants with tricyclic antidepressants may enhance the activity of both substances.

## Clinical Pearls

- The use of atomoxetine is suggested in children and adolescents who cannot tolerate stimulants.

- It may also be helpful for those with significant anxiety that may be exacerbated by stimulants.

# Psychotherapeutic and Psychosocial Interventions

# 29 Planning for Psychotherapeutic Interventions

## Clinical Snapshot

Jane is a 14-year-old girl that you've known since birth. A wide-eyed, curious, intelligent child all her life, she has had no major medical issues in the years that you have been treating her. Since starting her new school, her levelheaded mother has been calling you for the past few months to voice some concerns. She is increasingly more alarmed by the changes she has seen in Jane.

Mom has noted that Jane is more mysterious, more irritable, and increasingly more moody and argumentative. This is a change they were expecting as Jane reached her teenage years, but it seems more intense than their experience with Jane's older sister. She has changed her clothing and music preferences – choosing darker colors and louder emo bands. She has also traded in her lifelong friends for kids that are into drugs, defiance, and rage.

Mom notes that Jane has been wearing long sleeves and pants even as the weather has gotten warmer. When she finally got a glimpse of Jane's arms yesterday, she saw 15 to 20 angry red scratches along her left forearm. When she confronted Jane, they argued to the point where Jane ran out of the house. She was out for a few hours and returned after midnight. Mom wonders what to do and asks for your professional opinion.

As the scenario above illustrates, there may be times when a child's needs exceed what your practice is able to comprehensively provide. At these times, referral to a mental health provider may not only be helpful, but also quite necessary. Psychotherapeutic intervention can be a powerful and effective tool for your patients and their families. Families will often call upon you, the provider who has known their child the longest, to provide referrals and information. Unfortunately, navigating the mental health system to find quality treatment can be difficult for families, particularly when they are in crisis. Your guidance and support is most crucial in these times to ensure that they get connected to the appropriate mental health providers who can work with you in helping the child and family.

## Where do I even begin to search for a mental health treatment provider?

Usually the best sources to locate a therapist are:
- Child and adolescent psychiatrists are the ideal physician specialists to whom you can refer such patients and families. They are the only providers who can provide you with a comprehensive treatment plan including suggestions for individual, group, and family therapy in addition to medication evaluations. Unfortunately, due to current severe shortage of child and adolescent psychiatrists, it may be difficult to find one in your area who is accepting new patients. If there are any in the community,

consider creating a consultative relationship where they would provide you with comprehensive evaluations and you may continue providing treatment for more straightforward cases.

- There are a number of excellent collaborative programs nationally where mental health services are co-located or work together with pediatricians and PCPs. The Massachusetts Child Psychiatry Access Project (MCPAP), for example, has set up 6 mental health teams to provide services statewide. Each team includes child and adolescent psychiatrists, therapists, and a care coordinator – all of whom are led by child and adolescent psychiatry divisions of academic medical centers, including Baystate Medical Center, Massachusetts General Hospital, and Children's Hospital Boston. Pediatricians and PCPs can access services such as telephone consultation, psychiatric/diagnostic evaluation, care coordination, psychotherapy, and local educational programming. MCPAP currently covers 1.5 million children and adolescents in the state. Consider contacting your local American Academy of Child and Adolescent Psychiatry regional organization (www.aacap.org) or American Academy of Pediatrics chapter (www.aap.org) to find out if such programs are available in your area.

- Contact your local community mental health centers – Many states have a network of community mental health centers that serve a particular geographic area. Talking to their intake department or crisis service may be helpful.

- Contact the child and adolescent psychiatry department at your local hospital or academic medical center. Establishing a relationship with specific providers can sometimes work better than utilizing intake departments. However, in case they do not have availability, intake departments usually keep a list of referrals which you can ask them to send you.

- One of the first places to look should be the insurance company list of providers. Unfortunately, our experience has been that many parents have often exhausted this list before coming to their pediatrician or PCP looking for help. They usually complain that the provider lists are either outdated or inadequate (for example, the only available provider is miles away or the first available appointment is months away). Insurers must provide access to providers if it is a covered benefit. Requesting that the insurer facilitate a single case agreement with a local out-of-network provider can be helpful. In certain states, contacting your state's insurance commission can often help to open doors to treatment for your patients.

- Depending on your geographic location, universities, teaching hospitals, and research departments may be conducting studies for which kids or families may qualify.

- Also consider looking into professional schools and residency training programs for social work, psychology, and psychiatry trainees.

- Most importantly, if you find someone good, develop and maintain that relationship. Also, even if the person is too busy to accept many new patients, ask them to come to your office to provide an educational in-service training session for you and your staff. There are many ways to reap the benefits of a good professional, but a relationship needs to be there.

## What makes for a qualified mental health practitioner? What should I be looking for?

Here are some key points to inquire about when attempting to locate the best provider for your patients:
- **What are the credentialing and licensing of the practitioner?** Psychotherapy can be provided by a range of credentialed clinicians. Credentials can include: medical doctors (MD) and doctors of

osteopathic medicine (DO); doctorates of philosophy (PhD) or psychology (PsyD) – usually these practitioners are clinical psychologists, though there are clinicians with doctorates in social work, education, and other related fields, and practitioners with masters-level degrees in social work (MSW), psychology, education (MEd), and nursing (MSN). Considering a practitioner's field of study can give you insight into the "lens" with which they may work with your patient. For example, a social worker would consider the impact of the various systems that your patient interfaces with in daily life. All practitioners should have valid licenses to practice in their fields. You can obtain information about current licensing through your state's department of health or licensing board. Specific license titles can vary from state to state. For example, some of these can include: licensed independent clinical social worker (LICSW) or licensed clinical social worker (LCSW); licensed mental health counselor (LMHC) and licensed marriage and family therapist (LMFT) for masters or doctoral level clinicians; advanced practice registered nurses (APRN) for masters level nurses; and licensed chemical dependency practitioner (LCDP) for master level substance abuse clinicians. There are other types of licenses, so check with your state licensing board to figure out which types of licensed providers exist in your community.

- **What is the practitioner's theoretical framework?** In order to provide your patient with care that suits their particular needs, it is important to consider the mental health provider's theoretical perspective. Below are a few of the possible frameworks:

  - Cognitive behavioral therapy (CBT) is a structured theoretical framework which focuses on exploring and changing a person's negative thought patterns to promote a decrease in maladaptive behaviors. CBT has been used successfully in working with patients struggling with depression, anxiety, and obsessive compulsive disorder (OCD).

  - Dialectical behavioral therapy (DBT) is a combination of CBT practices and mindfulness tenets of Zen philosophy to help patients struggling with emotion regulation, interpersonal relatedness, and distress tolerance. An evidence-based practice, it has been adapted for a wide range of populations including adolescents struggling with depression, personality issues, and anxiety.

  - In both CBT and DBT, there is usually a time limit to the therapy relationship, a set structure for sessions, homework assignments, and skills to be practiced between meetings.

  - Psychodynamic theory is a framework that takes into consideration conscious and subconscious content during sessions, as well as focusing on the relationship between the patient and therapist. There is usually no set structure to these sessions and to the length of time a therapy relationship can continue. This framework is also effective with many psychiatric disorders.

  - All of the mentioned theoretical frameworks can be delivered within a wide range of modalities, examples of which are discussed next.

- **What modality does the practitioner provide?** There are four major of modalities that clinicians can use depending on what is occurring for the child or within the family.

  - **Individual Therapy:** Many of your patients will be able to benefit from individual therapy, which can be used to help youths to understand their actions and thoughts in an attempt to help them gain better control over their thoughts or behaviors. Some patients may be having difficulty because they don't know how to talk about strong emotions, have coped with emotions by using maladaptive behaviors, or need to learn more effective coping skills. Individual therapy is also beneficial in cases where children are self-harming, have eating disorders, are experiencing parental divorce, or are abused or neglected.

  - **Family Therapy:** Remember, kids live within families; this relationship is transactional and dynamic. Family therapy focuses on exploring maladaptive communication patterns. Examples of

situations where family therapy may be helpful are with kids who are unable or unwilling to follow their parent's rules or expectations, parents who are inconsistent with limit setting, kids with
eating disorders, and those having difficulties with school. Family therapy can also be useful when
families are in need of psychoeducation around their child's diagnoses or to help them understand
the psychological changes occurring to a family member.

- **Group Therapy:** Some patients benefit from group therapy. The goal of groups is to provide a safe,
comfortable environment where peers are able to provide feedback and insight to one another on
emotional issues. It can also provide patients with the experience that they are not the only person
struggling with an issue. Youths who usually benefit the most from such groups are those who have
experienced a loss, those struggling with social skills, emotion regulation, or anger management
issues.

- **Couples Therapy:** Lastly, parents who are having difficulty getting along or are unable to coparent
effectively could benefit from couples therapy. Sometimes, couples therapy may be helpful because
their child's difficulties are straining the parent's relationship. It is not advisable to have divorced
parents attend couples therapy – it is better for them to get on the same page by attending joint
meetings or family therapy sessions.

• **What is the practitioner's area(s) of specialty or interest?** In certain situations you may find that
your patient needs a more specialized type of therapy. These can include, but are not limited to, those
who have experienced a trauma, are struggling with eating disorders, substance dependency, and
adoption or attachment issues. Ideally the therapist you refer your patient to has a knowledge base
compatible to the kid's issues.

• **How often can the practitioner see the child and/or family?** This is a very important consideration.
If your patient is exhibiting risky behaviors, has experienced recent trauma, is emotionally labile, or
is demonstrating impulsive behaviors you will want a therapist with the flexibility to see your patient
weekly, and to have availability to see the child unexpectedly. Most clinicians will be able to provide
this service. Some clinicians only schedule time to see their clients every other week or monthly.
Those clinicians are better suited for kids who are more stable and require "maintenance" or supportive therapy.

## Are there things which are patient or family specific in order to find the right fit?

There are other issues to consider that can increase the likelihood of finding a good match for your patient.
The better you can meet their needs, the greater the probability that they remain committed to treatment
and that their parents feel progress is being made. Additional things to consider when helping to find a
therapist are:

• **Gender of the practitioner.** Some kids and teens prefer the familiarity of a same-gendered clinician.
Others prefer someone who is the opposite gender, particularly if they are lacking a strong same-
gendered role model or when this relationship is challenging. This may be an issue for kids who have
had traumatic or abusive experiences, and particularly for teens, who may feel more comfortable talking about issues of sexuality to a person of their same gender. Having a conversation with the patient
or parent about this can be helpful.

• **Age and experience of the practitioner.** From a developmental perspective, teens may not trust the
intentions of adults or may not believe that adults have had experiences similar to theirs. A younger
clinician may be able to traverse the "generation gap" more effectively than an older colleague, and
could offer a fresh perspective and energy to your patient. Also, younger or less experienced clinicians

are more likely to be involved in supervisory relationships to help them refine techniques and work through issues that may arise in sessions. However, with age usually comes experience, and seasoned clinicians may have more "tools" for working with kids and families. They may be more likely to tolerate the nonlinear process of change without over-reacting in a potential crisis. Of course, parents are usually more put at ease by a more experienced clinician.

- **Ethnicity, race, or culture of the child and practitioner.** A culturally compatible (or at least culturally competent) clinician is more likely to speak your patient's language, avoiding the need for involving an interpreter. They could better establish rapport and trust with the family, possibly allowing for increased disclosure of information, for feeling valued and understood by their provider, and for remaining connected to therapy. One possible pitfall of matching a patient and their clinician culturally is that the common "shorthand" used within the culture may lead a clinician to overlook important issues.

- **Size of the clinician's practice.** Does the clinician work within a small private practice or as part of a larger mental health agency? Patients will have access to more intensive levels of care (including intensive outpatient and day programs), auxiliary services, and a formal protocol for handling crises at a larger mental health agency. Private practitioners are usually more seasoned clinicians as some states require a more advanced license to practice privately. Assessment of your patient's needs should dictate where you send your patients for care.

- **Style of the practitioner.** Teens will often say that they want a counselor to interact with them instead of sitting quietly and nodding. Then again, other teens complain that their therapist was trying too hard to be their peer or friend, which can also feel "weird." Understand what your patient would like. A good style match between patient and provider increases the rapport building opportunities with the child and family. This can help to secure a commitment to treatment.

- **Should there be multiple practitioners involved with the child and family?** There are times when it makes clinical sense to arrange for separate therapists to provide individual and family therapy. This is developmentally appropriate for teens, who may prefer their own person to confide in separate from the family clinician, who may be seen as allied with the parents.

- **Insurance and funding issues.** With higher copays for mental health services as well as annual limits on mental health visits, mental health treatment can be costly for families. Having an idea of what a family's behavioral health benefits are before making a referral for care is essential. Assessing the family's ability to pay out-of-pocket for treatment may also open more opportunities for them to be seen by a private practitioner.

One common analogy used to describe the referral process is: "Finding a good therapist is like finding a great pair of jeans. It can take trying on lots of different styles, but don't get discouraged. Once you find the best pair, you'll settle into their comforts and forget about the trials of finding them." Throughout the referral process and in the earliest stages of treatment, it is important to remind kids and families (and yourself) that therapy is not a "magical process," forward progress takes time and there may be a need to try different practitioners to find the best match. It may be helpful to assist your patient and family make small, time-limited commitments to treatment instead of thinking about it as a never-ending relationship. Suggest that they commit to ten sessions with their therapist, follow up with them often and review how things are progressing so they don't feel like they have fallen into an abyss with no way out. Encourage families and especially adolescents to take note of their first impressions of their new therapist, but challenge them to keep an open mind to the possibility that this impression could change over time. Finally, if they bring concerns to you about how the work is progressing, remind them that therapists are professionals who need feedback from their patients to know if they are making good progress; a good therapist will modify the interactional style to meet patients where they are or refer them elsewhere if they cannot meet their needs. Feedback, both positive and negative, is encouraged and expected.

# 30 Planning for Psychosocial Interventions

*There is a vitality, a life force, an energy, a quickening,
that is translated through you into action, and because
there is only one of you in all time, this expression is
unique. And if you block it, it will never exist through any
other medium and will be lost.*
Martha Graham (1894–1991)

Why must everything be about what's wrong and how to treat it? Isn't there something to be said for an old fashioned baseball game in the neighborhood sand lot, organized for kids by kids, with parents at home content that their children are having a good time? And that if a neighbor down the street saw them doing anything else, wouldn't they call with an update? The times are changing and this scene is one that rarely seems to play out today.

However, the fundamental question that needs to be asked is whether a clinical model of pathology, etiology, and treatment has room for alternative ways of providing support to kids and families based on a child's *strengths, talents, and interests*? Psychosocial supports are essential to provide kids with a well-rounded experience of childhood and to offer them, and their parents, a renewed sense of social awareness and community. For many youths dealing with mental health issues, it is this isolation from their peers and the feeling of being left out of something bigger that is perhaps the hardest pill to swallow. It is important – when developing a treatment plan for the child in your office who may be depressed, or have a learning disorder, or have poor self-worth – to think beyond the diagnosis to the actual child and family.

As much as it is important to find the right medication or refer them to the right therapist, sometimes the most helpful thing that you can do is to thoughtfully consider the psychosocial interventions that you can help to put into place. For example, for the child who is presenting to your office due to poor academic performance and possible ADHD symptoms, your involvement and advocacy on the child's behalf could make a significant impact by ensuring that an appropriate 504 plan or individualized educational plan (IEP) is instated. Likewise, for the child who is shy and depressed, who tends to isolate in the bedroom for hours at a time, suggested involvement in a local Girl Scout troop or joining the local YMCA may open a world of new experiences. Involvement in community activities allows kids to be able to practice social skills and have more real-life, proximal supports. This can reduce the likelihood of reliance on video games, television, and the Internet for social contact and entertainment. Additionally, these community experiences can provide valuable information that can be used in therapy sessions; successes can be praised, and challenges can be explored for alternative ways to handle a situation. Children who see their relationship with the community as reciprocal may be more likely to feel an increased responsibility to it and be less likely to jeopardize their role in it.

Regardless of the patient's chief complaint, think about the needs of the child. What would help this child to do better? What are the readily accessible community supports that can help this child? How much more can we accomplish for this child by thinking out of the box and from looking at the child without a disease-oriented pathologizing perspective?

Trying to find psychosocial supports can be equally as challenging for families as finding a good therapist. They may ask you for advice and suggestions. As always, the first thing to do is to assess what your patient's areas of strengths and deficits are, what they like to do, have done in the past and their level of comfort with social situations. A shy child with motor skills deficits may not be the ideal candidate for a team sport, but could excel in martial arts classes where the focus is on individual achievement within a group learning environment. Communicating with school personnel can be helpful in assessing your patient's attention span, social skills, and ability to respond to authority as well as their academic progress. Local parent support groups and informational websites can offer additional resources.

Playing on a soccer team or joining a recreational club can provide a child with hands-on learning experience that can enhance self-esteem and offer a glimpse of what they can accomplish. Common areas to look for psychosocial supports include, but are not limited to, YMCA's, Boys and Girls Clubs, and other youth recreational clubs. Churches, synagogues, temples, and other places of worship may have youth groups and recreational activities that your patient can join. Structured activities such as martial arts training, arts and crafts classes, yoga and exercise classes, and camp may be other resources.

Older adolescents can also be encouraged to look for jobs or volunteer opportunities at local hospitals, animal shelters, and food banks. Although there may be the need for guidance and supervision by the parents to make sure they are responsible and emotionally capable enough to maintain both a job and expected achievement levels at school, this can be a great opportunity to show that they are maturing and can be more responsible.

If a child is not able to participate in community activities that typically developing peers experience due to behavioral or emotional outbursts, there are other options to consider for them. To help them experience supportive community programming, mental health agencies often have listings of therapeutic recreational programming. These offerings often have fun activities with a supportive clinical piece involved. Children's Hospital Boston, for example, offered a very popular therapeutic basketball group for kids with autism spectrum disorders who otherwise could not participate in activities that require joint attention and significant social and communication skills. Big Brothers, Big Sisters, and other mentoring programs can provide strong role models for at-risk youth. Finally, parents can find information about education and support groups on approved websites for children and adolescents struggling with mental health issues, such as the National Alliance for the Mentally Ill (www.nami.org) and the American Academy of Child and Adolescent Psychiatry (www.aacap.org).

As much as we want to help kids, it is also important to meet the needs of parents. Respite services may be offered by local community and religious organizations. Parent support groups can be helpful to allow parents to support each other. Local educational talks, such as the Parenting Matters series at Bradley Hospital, are excellent ways for parents to get more information in a nonthreatening environment.

As you start finding different resources in your community, start making a list and provide it to children and families. Contact local organizations and find out whether they already have lists of their own that they can share with you. Also, local community mental health centers and mental health providers may have additional information as well.

When working with a family in crisis, it is important to think about supporting the patient and the family with psychosocial supports. The better the support system that can be developed, the more successful they can be.

> *"You can discover more about a person in an hour of play*
> *than in a year of conversation."*
> Plato (427 BC–347 BC)

# Appendices

This section reviews the following materials:

- Appendix A – Comprehensive Psychiatric Evaluation
- Appendix B – Suicide and Risk Assessment
- Appendix C – Concise Overview of Pertinent DSM-IV-TR Diagnoses
- Appendix D – Commonly Used DSM-IV-TR Diagnostic Codes
- Appendix E – Suggested Rating Scales
- Appendix F – References and Sources for Additional Information

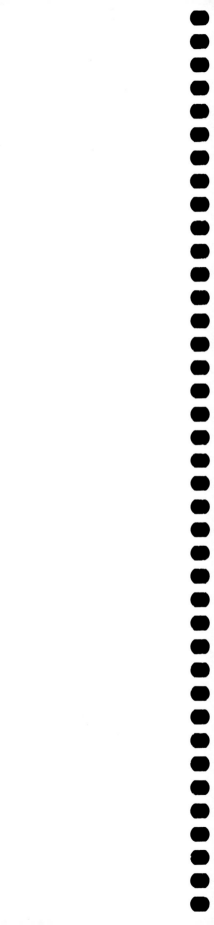

# Appendix A:
# Comprehensive Psychiatric Evaluation

## Comprehensive Psychiatric Evaluation*

Name:
DOB:
MR #:

| Assessment Date: | | Time: | |
|---|---|---|---|
| **Informant Name** | | **Relationship** | **Phone** |
| | | | |
| | | | |

Additional Sources of Information:

**Chief Complaint:**

**History of Present Illness:**

<br>
<br>
<br>
<br>
<br>

**Appetite** ☐ developmentally appropriate ☐ excessive ☐ increased ☐ decreased ☐ other:

**Energy/Libido** ☐ developmentally appropriate ☐ increased ☐ decreased ☐ other:

**Sleep** ☐ unremarkable ☐ hypersomnia ☐ insomnia: ☐ initial ☐ middle ☐ early awakening ☐ other:

**Weight** ☐ unremarkable ☐ loss 1–10 lbs ☐ loss 10+ lbs ☐ gain 1–10 lbs ☐ gain 10+ lbs ☐ other:

**Current Suicidal Ideation?** ☐ no ☐ yes    **Intent?** ☐ no ☐ yes    **Plan?** ☐ no ☐ yes

**Current Homicidial Ideation?** ☐ no ☐ yes    **Intent?** ☐ no ☐ yes    **Plan?** ☐ no ☐ yes

**Imminent Danger to Self?** ☐ no ☐ yes

**Imminent Danger to Others?** ☐ no ☐ yes

*(If yes for any of the above items, complete Appendix B - Suicide and Risk Assessment Form)*

**Past Psychiatric History:** (Include dates, reason, type of treatment, and reasons for discontinuing)    ☐ **none**

<br>
<br>
<br>

**Past Medical/Surgical History:**    ☐ **none**

<br>
<br>

**Past Psychiatric Medications:**    ☐ **none**

<br>
<br>

**Current Treatment?** ☐ no ☐ yes, Provider:      Telephone:

Treatment Type:      Date Last Seen:

\* Adapted by Dr. Trivedi from the Initial Evaluation Report of the Bradley Hospital.

This page may be reproduced by the purchaser for clinical use. All rights reserved.
From: Trivedi HK, Kershner JD: *Practical Child and Adolescent Psychiatry for Pediatrics and Primary Care*    © 2009 Hogrefe & Huber Publishers

## Comprehensive Psychiatric Evaluation*

Name:
DOB:
MR #:

| Medications: ☐ unavailable ☐ **none** | | Pharmacy: Tel: | | |
|---|---|---|---|---|
| C* | Medication/Dose/Frequency | Reason | Last Dose | Compliant |
| | | | | |
| | | | | |
| | | | | |
| | | | | |
| | | | | |
| | | | | |

C* = confirmed by: ☐ pharmacy ☐ medication bottle ☐ prescriber ☐ parent

| **Allergies/Medication Adverse Effects:** | | | | ☐ unavailable ☐ **NKA** |
|---|---|---|---|---|
| Category** | Allergen/Medication | Reaction | Treatment | Hx ER Visit? |
| ☐ A ☐ AE | | | | ☐ Y ☐ N ☐ ? |
| ☐ A ☐ AE | | | | ☐ Y ☐ N ☐ ? |
| ☐ A ☐ AE | | | | ☐ Y ☐ N ☐ ? |
| ☐ A ☐ AE | | | | ☐ Y ☐ N ☐ ? |
| Comments: | | | | |

** A = allergy AE = adverse effect

| **Risk/Safety Assessment:** | | | | ☐ unavailable |
|---|---|---|---|---|
| **Behaviors** | No Hx | Active | Past Hx | Describe |
| Suicidal ideation/gestures | | | | |
| Homicidal ideation/gestures | | | | |
| Self-injurious behaviors | | | | |
| Aggression (identify targets) | | | | |
| Sexualized behavior | | | | |
| Access to guns | | | | |
| Legal issues | | | | |
| Other | | | | |

| **Trauma/Abuse History:** | | | | ☐ none |
|---|---|---|---|---|
| Type | N | Y | Description | Time Frame/Duration |
| Sexual abuse | | | | |
| Physical abuse | | | | |
| Neglect | | | | |
| Other trauma: | | | | |
| **Trauma associated symptoms present:** ☐ NONE ☐ nightmares ☐ intrusive thoughts ☐ avoidance | | | | |
| ☐ numbness, detachment ☐ hyper-vigilance, startling ☐ other: | | | | |
| Describe findings: | | | | |

* Adapted by Dr. Trivedi from the Initial Evaluation Report of the Bradley Hospital.

From: Trivedi HK, Kershner JD: *Practical Child and Adolescent Psychiatry for Pediatrics and Primary Care*    © 2009 Hogrefe & Huber Publishers

## Comprehensive Psychiatric Evaluation*

Name:
DOB:
MR #:

| Family Psychiatric History: | | | ☐ **none** |
|---|---|---|---|
| Relative | Diagnosis | Treatment | Tx Effective |
| | | | ☐ Y  ☐ N  ☐ ? |
| | | | ☐ Y  ☐ N  ☐ ? |

Family History of Suicide?  ☐ no  ☐ yes

Family History of Substance Abuse?  ☐ no  ☐ yes

**Social History:**

Substance History:

Sexual History:

Lives With:

Parents Employment:

Parents Marital Status:

Family Stressors:

Agency Involvement:  ☐ none  ☐ DCYF/DSS  ☐ other:

School: Grade: IEP/504?  ☐ no  ☐ yes

Decline in academic performance?  ☐ no  ☐ yes

**Mental Status Examination**

Appearance:

**Behavior:**  ☐ calm  ☐ cooperative  ☐ guarded  ☐ suspicious  ☐ hostile  ☐ withdrawn  ☐ other:

**Motor:**  ☐ unremarkable  ☐ psychomotor agitation  ☐ psychomotor retardation  ☐ tics  ☐ tremors  ☐ abnormal movements  ☐ other/describe:

**Speech:**  ☐ unremarkable  ☐ abnormal rate  ☐ abnormal rhythm  ☐ abnormal volume  ☐ abnormal productivity  ☐ other/describe:

**Mood:**

**Affect:**  ☐ euthymic  ☐ dysphoric  ☐ labile  ☐ expansive  ☐ flat  ☐ blunted  ☐ constricted  ☐ mood congruent  ☐ appropriate  ☐ other/describe:

**Thought Process:**  ☐ linear  ☐ circumstantial  ☐ tangential  ☐ loose  ☐ flight of ideas  ☐ racing thoughts  ☐ blocking  ☐ slowed  ☐ other/describe:

**Thought Content:**  ☐ developmentally appropriate  ☐ hallucinations  ☐ delusions  ☐ suicidal  ☐ homicidal  ☐ obsessions  ☐ other/describe:

**Insight:**  ☐ developmentally appropriate  ☐ fair  ☐ poor  ☐ other:

**Judgment:**  ☐ developmentally appropriate  ☐ fair  ☐ poor  ☐ other:

**Impulse Control:**  ☐ adequate for interview  ☐ fair  ☐ poor  ☐ other:

**Insight:**  ☐ unremarkable  ☐ fair  ☐ poor  ☐ developmentally appropriate ☐ other:

\* Adapted by Dr. Trivedi from the Initial Evaluation Report of the Bradley Hospital.

From: Trivedi HK, Kershner JD: *Practical Child and Adolescent Psychiatry for Pediatrics and Primary Care*      © 2009 Hogrefe & Huber Publishers

## Comprehensive Psychiatric Evaluation*

Name:
DOB:
MR #:

### Cognitive Functioning

| | correct | incorrect | NA* | UA* | | correct | incorrect | NA* | UA* |
|---|---|---|---|---|---|---|---|---|---|
| Day | ☐ | ☐ | ☐ | ☐ | Immediate Recall 3/3 | ☐ | ☐ | ☐ | ☐ |
| Date | ☐ | ☐ | ☐ | ☐ | 5 Minute Recall | ☐ | ☐ | ☐ | ☐ |
| Time | ☐ | ☐ | ☐ | ☐ | Current Events | ☐ | ☐ | ☐ | ☐ |
| Place | ☐ | ☐ | ☐ | ☐ | WORLD | ☐ | ☐ | ☐ | ☐ |
| Person | ☐ | ☐ | ☐ | ☐ | DLROW | ☐ | ☐ | ☐ | ☐ |
| Proverbs | ☐ | ☐ | ☐ | ☐ | Serial 7's or 3's | ☐ | ☐ | ☐ | ☐ |

NA* = not applicable UA* = unable to test

### Assessment

### Multi-Axial DSM Diagnoses

**Axis I:**

**Axis II:**

**Axis III:**

**Axis IV:** ☐ none ☐ primary support group ☐ social environment ☐ education ☐ occupation ☐ housing ☐ financial ☐ access to health care ☐ legal issues ☐ other/describe:

**Axis V (GAF):** current: highest in past year:

### Plan

**Treatment plan discussed with patient, parent/legal guardian:** ☐ yes ☐ no, explain:

| Signature: | Date: |
|---|---|
| Print Name: | Time: |

* Adapted by Dr. Trivedi from the Initial Evaluation Report of the Bradley Hospital.

# Appendix B:
# Suicide and Risk Assessment

## Suicide and Risk Assessment*

Name:
DOB:
MR #:

| Date of Assessment: | Time of Assessment: | Parent/Guardian Present: ☐ yes ☐ no | | |
|---|---|---|---|---|
| **History of Suicide Attempt(s)?** ☐ no ☐ yes, details listed below. | | | | |
| Total # Attempts: Date of First Attempt? Most Recent Attempt? | | **Risk Factors** | **Y** | **N** |
| Description of Event(s) and Method(s) Used: | | Lethal Means? | | |
| | | Low Probability of Rescue? | | |
| | | Planned Attempt? | | |
| Trigger(s): | | Expressed Intent to Die? | | |
| | | Remorseful About Attempt? | | |
| **History of Self-Injurious Behavior(s)?** ☐ no ☐ yes, details listed below. | | | | |
| Self-Cutting? Needed Stitches? Superficial Scratches? Head Banging? Self-Choking? Self-Burning? | | | | |
| Total # Attempts: | Date of First Attempt? | Most Recent Attempt? | | |
| Description of Event(s) and Method(s) Used: | | | | |
| | | | | |
| Trigger(s): | | | | |
| | | | | |
| **History of Risky or Reckless Behavior?** ☐ no ☐ yes, details listed below. | | | | |
| Total # Attempts: | Date of First Attempt? | Most Recent Attempt? | | |
| Description of Event(s): | | | | |
| | | | | |
| Trigger(s): | | | | |
| Substance Use? ☐ no ☐ yes, describe: | | | | |
| Aggression, Theft, or Risky Sexual Behaviors? ☐ no ☐ yes, describe: | | | | |
| Legal Issues? ☐ no ☐ yes, describe: | | | | |
| Sustained Harm or Injury to Self? ☐ no ☐ yes, describe: | | | | |
| Harm or Injury to Peers? ☐ no ☐ yes, describe: | | | | |
| Potential for Serious Harm to Self or Others? ☐ no ☐ yes, describe: | | | | |
| **Suicidal Ideation** | | | | |
| Have you ever felt that it would be okay if you went to sleep and did not wake up? | | ☐ no ☐ **current ☐ **past | | |
| Do you ever feel that it might be better if you weren't alive any more? | | ☐ no ☐ **current ☐ **past | | |
| Have you ever had thoughts of wanting to be dead or even trying to kill yourself? | | ☐ no ☐ **current ☐ **past | | |
| Have you ever gotten to the point that you had the intention of killing yourself? | | ☐ no ☐ **current ☐ **past | | |
| Have you ever thought about how you might do this? | | ☐ no ☐ **current ☐ **past | | |
| Have you ever bought or obtained things necessary to end your life? | | ☐ no ☐ **current ☐ **past | | |
| Have you ever written good-bye letters or made preparations for your death? | | ☐ no ☐ **current ☐ **past | | |
| **Details (description of events and triggers): | | | | |
| | | | | |

| Suicide and Risk Assessment* | Name:<br>DOB:<br>MR #: |
|---|---|

### Intensity of Current Suicidal Ideation *(if suicidal ideation present)*

How often have you had these thoughts in the past week? □ < 1× /wk  □ 1× /wk  □ 2–5× /wk  □ daily  □ many × /d

When you had these thoughts, how long did they last? □ fleeting/few minutes  □ few hours □ most of the day □ persistently

Have you thought about how you would hurt yourself? □ no  □ yes, describe:

Right now, do you feel like you want to hurt yourself  □ no  □ yes, describe:

Do you have access to firearms or any other lethal means? □ no  □ yes, describe:

### Risk Factors

| Diagnostic | Y | N | Demographic | Y | N | Stressors | Y | N | Biopsychosocial | Y | N |
|---|---|---|---|---|---|---|---|---|---|---|---|
| Mood Disorder | | | Male Sex | | | Recent Significant Loss | | | Fam History Suicide | | |
| Substance Abuse | | | Adolescent | | | Peer Suicide / Death | | | Impulsivity | | |
| Psychosis | | | Caucasian | | | Relationship Break-Up | | | Poor coping skills | | |
| | | | Native American | | | History Abuse / Neglect | | | Poor self-regulation | | |

### Protective Factors

| Social Environment | Y | N | Therapeutic Alliance | Y | N |
|---|---|---|---|---|---|
| Supportive Family | | | Intact Therapeutic Alliance | | |
| Competent Family | | | Actively Involved in Treatment | | |
| Friendship Network | | | Compliant with Recommendations / Follow-Up | | |

### Assessment of Suicidality and Risks (Also Include Description of Protective Factors)

### Plan

Parent/Guardian Aware of Current Risks/Concerns?  □ no  □ yes

Need for Acute Intervention?  □ no  □ yes

| Signature: | Date: |
|---|---|
| Print Name: | Time: |

* Adapted by Dr. Trivedi from the Initial Evaluation Report of the Bradley Hospital.

From: Trivedi HK, Kershner JD: *Practical Child and Adolescent Psychiatry for Pediatrics and Primary Care*   © 2009 Hogrefe & Huber Publishers

# Appendix C:
# Concise Overview of Pertinent DSM-IV-TR Diagnoses*

This appendix reviews the pertinent DSM-IV-TR diagnoses that you are more likely to use routinely. The information is presented more so as a quick reference to jog your memory about particular diagnoses. For example, when you are interacting with a patient or family and can't remember what Bipolar II Disorder is, this is a helpful place to get some additional information. The text and tables below do <u>not</u> represent all of the criteria needed to make a diagnosis and cross-referencing with the DSM-IV-TR is suggested. Diagnoses are clustered by type for easier searching and are listed in order of appearance in the DSM-IV-TR. For example, all mood disorders are listed together. When using the DSM for diagnosis it is often just as important to know why someone does not meet criteria for a particular diagnosis as much as it is important for them to fully meet the diagnosis. Please note that this list does not include all diagnoses, as it focuses on commonly used diagnoses for children and adolescents.

## Disorders Usually First Diagnosed in Infancy, Childhood, or Adolescence

### Mental Retardation

| Severity | IQ |
|---|---|
| Mild | 50–55 to 70 |
| Moderate | 35–40 to 50–55 |
| Severe | 20–25 to 35–40 |
| Profound | < 20–25 |

## Pervasive Developmental Disorders

### Autistic Disorder

- Onset before 3 years of age
- Deficiencies in social interaction, communication, and presence of restrictive/stereotyped behaviors
  - *Social Interaction:*
    - Decreased nonverbal behavior (eye-to-eye gage)
    - Decreased peer relationships
    - Decreased social or emotional reciprocity
  - *Communication:*
    - Decreased speech
    - Decreased conversational ability
    - Use of repetitive language
    - Decreased play (make believe or social)

* Adapted from: American Psychiatric Association. *Diagnostic and Statistical Manual of Mental Disorders DSM-IV-TR.* Washington DC: American Psychiatric Publishing, Inc.; 2000. DSM-IV-TR is a registered trademark of the American Psychiatric Association.

- *Restrictive/Stereotyped Behavior:*
    - Inflexible adherence to routines
    - Repetitive motor mannerisms
    - Preoccupation with parts of objects

### Asperger's Disorder

- Presence of deficiencies in social interaction
- Presence of restrictive/stereotyped behaviors
- No deficiency in language development

### Rett's Disorder

- Normal development through first 5 months after birth
- Normal head circumference at birth
- Loss of motor skills and deceleration of head growth after 5 months old

### Childhood Disintegrative Disorder

- Apparently normal development for first two years of life
- Developing deficiencies in social interaction, communication, or presence of restrictive/stereotyped behaviors
- Loss of previously acquired skills

### Pervasive Developmental Disorder Not Otherwise Specified

- Not meeting full criteria of any of the above diagnoses

## Attention Deficit and Disruptive Behavior Disorders

### Attention Deficit Hyperactivity Disorder (ADHD)

- Inattention symptoms for greater than 6 months
- Hyperactivity-impulsivity symptoms for greater than 6 months
- Some of the symptoms present before 7 years of age
- Symptoms occur in 2 or more settings

### Conduct Disorder

- Repetitive pattern of behavior violating basic rights of others or societal norms
    - Aggression to people and animals
    - Destruction of property

- Deceitfulness or theft
- Serious violations of rules
- If greater than 18 years old, consider whether Antisocial Personality Disorder

### Oppositional Defiant Disorder

- Negativistic, hostile, and defiant behavior

## Tic Disorders

### Tourette's Disorder

- Repetitive motor and vocal tics
- Never tic-free for more than 3 months
- Onset before 18 years of age

## Elimination Disorders

### Encopresis

- Repeated passage of feces in inappropriate places
- At least once per month for 3 months
- At least 4 years of age

### Enuresis

- Repeated voiding of urine into bed or clothes
- Twice weekly for three months or impacts functioning
- At least 5 years of age

## Other Disorders of Infancy, Childhood, or Adolescence

### Separation Anxiety Disorder

- Excessive anxiety on separation from home or loved ones
- Onset before 18 years of age
- Lasting greater than 4 weeks

*Selective Mutism*

- Consistent failure to speak in specific social situations despite speaking in others
- Symptoms for greater than a month (not only first month at school)

*Reactive Attachment Disorder of Infancy or Early Childhood*

- Disturbed or inappropriate social relatedness in most contexts
- Onset before age 5
- Presence of pathogenic care

# Delirium, Dementia, and Amnestic and Other Cognitive Disorders

*Delirium*

- Disturbance of consciousness with change in cognition or development of perceptual disturbance
- Disturbance develops over a short time and tends to fluctuate through the course of a day

# Substance-Related Disorders

*Substance Abuse*

- Recurrent use leading to failure to meet obligations at work, school, or home
- Recurrent use in dangerous situations
- Recurrent substance related legal issues
- Recurrent use despite interpersonal difficulties

*Substance Dependence*

- Development of tolerance
- Development of withdrawal
- Inability to cut down use despite recurrent problems
- Significant time spent in obtaining, use, or sobering from the substance

*Substance Withdrawal*

- Withdrawal symptoms related to stopping or decreasing use of that substance after period of significant use

## Polysubstance Dependence

- Using three or more groups of substances within past year
- No single substance was predominant

| | Intoxication | Withdrawal |
|---|---|---|
| **Alcohol** | – Slurred speech<br>– Incoordination<br>– Unsteady gait<br>– Nystagmus<br>– Impaired attention or memory<br>– Stupor/coma | – Autonomic hyperactivity<br>– Increased hand tremor<br>– Insomnia<br>– Nausea or vomiting<br>– Transient visual, tactical, or auditory hallucinations<br>– Psychomotor agitation<br>– Anxiety<br>– Grand mal seizures |
| **Amphetamine** | – Tachycardia or bradycardia<br>– Pupillary dilation<br>– Elevated or lowered blood pressure<br>– Perspiration or chills<br>– Nausea or vomiting<br>– Psychomotor agitation or retardation<br>– Weight loss<br>– Muscle weakness, respiratory depression, chest pain or cardiac arrhythmias | – Dysphoric mood<br>– Fatigue<br>– Vivid, unpleasant dreams<br>– Insomnia or hypersomnia<br>– Increased appetite<br>– Psychomotor agitation or retardation |
| **Caffeine (>250mg)** | – Restlessness<br>– GI disturbance<br>– Nervousness<br>– Muscle twitching<br>– Excitement<br>– Tachycardia<br>– Insomnia<br>– Inexhaustibility<br>– Flushed face<br>– Psychomotor agitation<br>– Diuresis<br>– Rambling thoughts or speech | None |
| **Cannabis** | – Symptoms within 2 hours<br>– Conjunctival injection<br>– Increased appetite<br>– Dry mouth<br>– Tachycardia | None |

|  | Intoxication | Withdrawal |
|---|---|---|
| **Cocaine** | - Tachycardia or bradycardia<br>- Pupillary dilation<br>- Elevated or lowered blood pressure<br>- Perspiration or chills<br>- Nausea or vomiting<br>- Psychomotor agitation or retardation<br>- Weight loss<br>- Muscle weakness, respiratory depression, chest pain or cardiac arrhythmias | - Dysphoric mood<br>- Fatigue<br>- Vivid, unpleasant dreams<br>- Insomnia or hypersomnia<br>- Increased appetite<br>- Psychomotor agitation or retardation |
| **Hallucinogen** | - Tachycardia<br>- Pupillary dilation<br>- Sweating<br>- Palpitations<br>- Blurred vision<br>- Tremors<br>- Incoordination | None |
| **Inhalant** | - Dizziness<br>- Nystagmus<br>- Incoordination<br>- Slurred speech<br>- Unsteady gait<br>- Lethargy<br>- Depressed reflexes<br>- Psychomotor retardation<br>- Tremor<br>- Blurred vision or diplopia<br>- Stupor or coma | None |
| **Nicotine** | - None | - Dysphoric or depressed mood<br>- Insomnia<br>- Irritability, frustration, or anger<br>- Anxiety<br>- Increased appetite or weight gain<br>- Difficulty concentrating<br>- Restlessness<br>- Decreased heart rate |
| **Opioids** | - Drowsiness or coma<br>- Slurred speech<br>- Impaired attention or memory | - Dysphoric mood<br>- Nausea or vomiting<br>- Muscle aches<br>- Lacrimation or rhinnorhea<br>- Diarrhea<br>- Yawning<br>- Pupillary dilation, piloerection, or sweating<br>- Fever<br>- Insomnia |

|  | Intoxication | Withdrawal |
|---|---|---|
| **Phencyclidine** | – Vertical or horizontal nystagmus<br>– Hypertension or tachycardia<br>– Decreased response to pain<br>– Ataxia<br>– Dysarthria<br>– Muscle rigidity<br>– Seizures<br>– Hyperacusis | None |
| **Sedative, Hypnotic, or Anxiolytic** | – Slurred speech<br>– Incoordination<br>– Unsteady gait<br>– Nystagmus<br>– Impaired attention or memory<br>– Stupor or coma | – Autonomic hyperactivity<br>– Increased hand tremor<br>– Insomnia<br>– Nausea or vomiting<br>– Transient visual, tactical, or auditory hallucinations<br>– Psychomotor agitation<br>– Anxiety<br>– Grand mal seizures |

# Schizophrenia and Other Psychotic Disorders

## Schizophrenia

- Delusions
- Hallucinations
- Disorganized speech
- Grossly disorganized or catatonic behavior
- Negative symptoms
- Symptoms for greater than 6 months
- Subtypes
    - Paranoid
    - Disorganized
    - Catatonic
    - Undifferentiated
    - Residual

## Schizophreniform Disorder

- Greater than 1 month, but less than 6 months of symptoms
- Symptom requirements similar to that for Schizophrenia
- Do not necessarily exhibit social or occupational dysfunction

### Brief Psychotic Disorder

- Greater than 1 day, but less than 1 month of symptoms
- Negative symptoms not part of decision

### Delusional Disorder

- Non-bizarre delusions for greater than 1 month
- Never met symptoms of Schizophrenia
- Functioning not markedly impaired

### Schizoaffective Disorder

- Depressive episode, manic episode, or mixed episode concurrent with schizophrenia symptoms
- Delusions or hallucinations for at least 2 weeks without mood symptoms

### Shared Psychotic Disorders

- Delusion develops in context of close relationship with another person who has the established delusion

## Mood Disorders

### Major Depressive Episode

- Either depressed mood (can be irritable mood in kids) or diminished interest/pleasure with impairment of functioning
- Weight loss (failure to make expected weight gain in kids)
- Insomnia or hypersomnia
- Psychomotor agitation or retardation
- Fatigue or loss of energy
- Worthlessness or excess guilt
- Decreased ability to think or concentrate
- Recurrent thoughts of death

### Manic Episode

- Elevated, expansive, or irritable mood
- Greater than 1 week of symptoms (or any duration if hospitalization needed)
- Inflated self-esteem or grandiosity
- Decreased need for sleep

- Pressured speech
- Flight of ideas or racing thoughts
- Distractibility
- Increased goal-directed activity or psychomotor agitation
- Excessive involvement in pleasurable activities with high potential for painful consequences
- Impaired social or occupational functioning

## Mixed Episode

- Criteria met for both Major Depressive Episode and Manic Episode for nearly every day in a 1 week period
- Impaired social or occupational functioning

## Hypomanic Episode

- Distinct period of persistently expansive or elevated mood for greater than 4 days which is different from usual mood
- Not severe enough to cause significant impairment

## Dysthymic Disorder

- Depressed mood most days for greater than 2 years (1 year in children and adolescents)
- Never a period of greater than 2 months without symptoms
- No depressive or manic episodes during first 2 years of disturbance

## Bipolar I Disorder

- Manic episodes with or without depressive ones

## Bipolar II Disorder

- Recurrent major depressive episodes with hypomanic episodes

## Cyclothymic Disorder

- Greater than 2 years of hypomanic symptoms with depressive symptoms not meeting criteria for MDD (1 year in kids)
- Not without symptoms for greater than 2 months
- No Major Depressive Episode, Manic Episode, or Mixed Episode in first 2 years

# Anxiety Disorders

## Panic Disorder

- Repeated panic attacks
- Palpitations
- Sweating
- Shaking
- Sensation of shortness of breath
- Choking feeling
- Chest pain
- Nausea
- Dizziness
- Derealization or depersonalization
- Fear of losing control or going crazy
- Paresthesias
- Chills or hot flashes
- 1 month of concern about additional attacks with worry about implications of the attack
- Indicate whether with or without agoraphobia

## Specific Phobia

- Exposure causes immediate anxiety
- Person realizes fear is unreasonable
- If patient older than 18 years, symptoms present for greater than 6 months

## Social Phobia

- Fear of social or performance situations
- Causes immediate anxiety
- Person realizes it is unreasonable
- Interferes with functioning
- If patient older than 18 years, symptoms last for greater than 6 months

## Obsessive-Compulsive Disorder

- Obsessions
    - Recurrent persistent intrusive or inappropriate thoughts, impulses, or images
    - Person realizes they are a product of their own mind

- Compulsions
  - Repetitive behaviors or mental acts that must be done to rigid rules to prevent or reduce distress
- Patient recognizes that they are excessive and unreasonable, except in young children
- Marked distress, taking greater than 1 hour/day, and interfering with their routine

### Posttraumatic Stress Disorder

- Exposed to traumatic event and responded with intense fear, helplessness, or horror (in kids, can be disorganized or agitated behavior)
- Event re-experienced by:
  - Recollections of event (repetitive play in kids)
  - Recurrent distressing dreams
  - Feeling as if traumatic event recurring
- Intense distress and physiological symptoms after exposure
- Avoidance of stimuli and numbing of general responsiveness
- Symptoms of increased arousal
- Symptoms lasting greater than 1 month

### Acute Stress Disorder

- Similar to PTSD above, but duration between 2 days and 4 weeks

### Generalized Anxiety Disorder

- Anxiety and excessive worry for most days in 6 months
- Difficult to control worry
- Associated with restlessness, easily fatigued, difficulty concentrating, irritability, muscle tension, and sleep disturbance
- Causes impairment of functioning

## Somatoform Disorders

### Somatization Disorder

- Multiple physical complaints before 30 years of age resulting in treatment being sought or impaired functioning
- 4 pain symptoms
- 2 gastrointestinal symptoms
- 1 sexual symptom

- 1 pseudoneurological symptom
- Symptoms not intentionally produced or feigned

### Conversion Disorder

- Psychological factors cause voluntary motor or sensory function symptoms or deficit
- Not intentionally produced

### Pain Disorder

- Psychological factors cause pain that impairs functioning
- Not intentionally produced

### Hypochondriasis

- Preoccupation with having a specific disease based on misinterpretation of bodily symptoms
- Continues despite appropriate medical evaluation
- Symptoms for greater than 6 months

### Body Dysmorphic Disorder

- Preoccupation with imagined defect in appearance
- Impairs functioning, causes distress

## Factitious Disorders

### Factitious Disorder

- Intentionally produced or feigning of symptoms
- Motivation to assume sick role

## Additional Conditions That May Be a Focus of Clinical Attention

### Malingering

- Intentional production or exaggeration of symptoms for external incentives

# Eating Disorders

## Anorexia Nervosa

- Refusal to maintain body weight (<85% of expected or failure to make expected gains)
- Fear of gaining weight or becoming fat
- Disturbance of body image
- Amennorhea
- Can be Restricting type or Binge-Eating/Purging Type

## Bulimia Nervosa

- Binge eating – lack of control over eating during episode
- Compensatory behavior such as use of laxatives or excessive exercise
- Occurs greater than twice weekly for 3 months
- Evaluation of self is influenced by body shape and weight
- Can be Purging Type or Non-Purging Type

# Sleep Disorders

### Primary Sleep Disorders

### Primary Insomnia

- Difficulty initiating or maintaining sleep for greater than 1 month

### Primary Hypersomnia

- Excessive sleepiness for greater than 1 month

### Narcolepsy

- Cataplexy and/or REM episodes occurring daily over greater than 3 months

### Breathing Related Sleep Disorder

- Breathing disruption related to breathing issue

### Circadian Rhythm Sleep Disorder

- Sleep disruption due to a mismatch between environmental sleep-wake cycle and circadian sleep-wake cycle

**Parasomnias**

*Nightmare Disorder*

- Repeatedly awakening with recollection of frightening dreams
- Quickly oriented and alert on waking
- Generally occurs during second half of sleep

*Sleep Terror Disorder*

- Repeatedly abrupt awakening from sleep
- Generally occurs during first third of sleep
- Intense autonomic arousal
- No detailed recollection of dream

*Sleepwalking Disorder*

- Rising from bed and walking
- Generally occurs during first third of sleep
- No memory of event

# Impulse Control Disorders

*Intermittent Explosive Disorder*

- Episodes of serious assaultive acts or property destruction

*Kleptomania*

- Repeatedly stealing objects not needed for personal use or monetary value
- Increasing tension before act and relief or gratification afterwards

*Pyromania*

- Deliberate and purposeful fire-setting
- Increasing tension before act and relief or gratification afterwards

*Trichotillomania*

- Repeatedly pulling out one's hair
- Increasing tension before act and relief or gratification afterwards

# Adjustment Disorders

*Adjustment Disorders*

- Emotional or behavioral symptoms
- In response to identifiable stressor within 3 months
- Marked distress and impairment
- Impairment in functioning
- Once stressor has terminated, symptoms do not persist for greater than 6 more months

# Appendix D:
# Commonly Used DSM-IV-TR Diagnostic Codes*

This appendix reviews the format for multi-axial diagnostic assessment. It also reviews DSM-IV-TR diagnostic codes that you are more likely to use routinely. Diagnoses are presented alphabetically for easier searching. To compare diagnoses within a diagnostic group, for example Major Depressive Disorder versus Depressive Disorder Not Otherwise Specified (NOS), please refer to the appropriate chapter in Section III of this text. Please note that this list does not include all diagnoses, as it focuses on commonly used diagnoses.

## Multi-Axial Diagnostic Assessment Format

- Axis I:      Clinical Disorders
- Axis II:     Personality Disorders and Mental Retardation
- Axis III:    General Medical Conditions
- Axis IV:     Psychosocial and Environmental Problems
- Axis V:      Global Assessment of Functioning

## Commonly Used DSM-IV-TR Codes

### A
| | |
|---|---|
| 308.3 | Acute Stress Disorder |
| ----- | Adjustment Disorder |
| 309.24 | – With Anxiety |
| 309.0 | – With Depressed Mood |
| 309.3 | – With Disturbance of Conduct |
| 309.28 | – With Mixed Anxiety and Depressed Mood |
| 309.4 | – With Mixed Disturbance of Emotions and Conduct |
| 309.9 | – Unspecified |
| 300.22 | Agoraphobia Without History of Panic Disorder |
| ----- | Alcohol |
| 305.00 | – Abuse |
| 303.90 | – Dependence |
| 303.00 | – Intoxication |
| 291.81 | – Withdrawal |
| ----- | Amphetamine |
| 305.70 | – Abuse |

* Adapted from: American Psychiatric Association. *Diagnostic and Statistical Manual of Mental Disorders DSM-IV-TR.* Washington DC: American Psychiatric Publishing, Inc.; 2000. DSM-IV-TR is a registered trademark of the American Psychiatric Association.

| 304.40 | – Dependence |
| 292.89 | – Intoxication |
| 292.81 | – Delirium |
| 292.0 | – Withdrawal |
| 307.1 | Anorexia Nervosa |
| ----- | Anxiety Disorder |
| 300.00 | – Anxiety Disorder NOS |
| 293.84 | – Due to...*[Indicate the General Medical Condition]* |
| 299.80 | Asperger's Disorder |
| ----- | Attention-Deficit/Hyperactivity Disorder |
| 314.9 | – Attention-Deficit/Hyperactivity Disorder NOS |
| 314.01 | – Combined Type |
| 314.01 | – Predominantly Hyperactive-Impulsive Type |
| 314.00 | – Predominantly Inattentive Type |
| 299.00 | Autistic Disorder |

# B

| 296.80 | Bipolar Disorder NOS |
| ----- | Bipolar I Disorder |
| 296.5x | – Most Recent Episode Depressed |
| | • *Specify Severity (×) = 1 Mild, 2 Moderate, 3 Severe, 4 Severe With Psychotic Features, 0 Unspecified* |
| 296.40 | – Most Recent Episode Hypomanic |
| 296.4x | – Most Recent Episode Manic |
| | • *Specify Severity (×) = 1 Mild, 2 Moderate, 3 Severe, 4 Severe With Psychotic Features, 0 Unspecified* |
| 296.6x | – Most Recent Episode Mixed |
| | • *Specify Severity (×) = 1 Mild, 2 Moderate, 3 Severe, 4 Severe With Psychotic Features, 0 Unspecified* |
| 296.7 | – Most Recent Episode Unspecified |
| 296.0x | – Single Manic Episode |
| | • *Specify Severity (×) = 1 Mild, 2 Moderate, 3 Severe, 4 Severe With Psychotic Features, 0 Unspecified* |
| 296.89 | Bipolar II Disorder |
| 298.8 | Brief Psychotic Disorder |
| 307.51 | Bulimia Nervosa |

# C

| ----- | Caffeine |
| 292.9 | – Caffeine-Related Disorder NOS |
| 305.90 | – Intoxication |
| ----- | Cannabis |
| 305.20 | – Abuse |
| 292.9 | – Cannabis-Related Disorder NOS |
| 304.30 | – Dependence |
| 292.89 | – Intoxication |
| 299.10 | Childhood Disintegrative Disorder |
| ----- | Cocaine |
| 305.60 | – Abuse |

| | | |
|---|---|---|
| 296.3x | – Recurrent | |
| | • *Specify Severity (×) = 1 Mild, 2 Moderate, 3 Severe,* | |
| | *4 Severe With Psychotic Features, 0 Unspecified* | |
| 296.2x | – Single Episode | |
| | • *Specify Severity (×) = 1 Mild, 2 Moderate, 3 Severe,* | |
| | *4 Severe With Psychotic Features, 0 Unspecified* | |
| ----- | Mental Retardation | |
| 317 | – Mild | |
| 318.0 | – Moderate | |
| 318.1 | – Severe | |
| 318.2 | – Profound | |
| 319 | – Severity Unspecified | |
| 293.83 | Mood Disorder Due to...*[Indicate the General Medical Condition]* | |
| 296.90 | Mood Disorder NOS | |

**N**

| | |
|---|---|
| ----- | Nicotine |
| 305.1 | – Dependence |
| 292.9 | – Nicotine-Related Disorder NOS |
| 292.0 | – Withdrawal |

**O**

| | |
|---|---|
| 300.3 | Obsessive-Compulsive Disorder |
| ----- | Opioid |
| 305.50 | – Abuse |
| 304.00 | – Dependence |
| 292.89 | – Intoxication |
| 292 | – Withdrawal |
| 313.81 | Oppositional Defiant Disorder |

**P**

| | |
|---|---|
| ----- | Pain Disorder |
| 307.80 | – Associated With Psychological Factors |
| 307.89 | – Associated With Both Psychological Factors and a General Medical Condition |
| ----- | Panic Disorder |
| 300.21 | – With Agoraphobia |
| 300.01 | – Without Agoraphobia |
| 299.80 | Pervasive Developmental Disorder NOS |
| ----- | Phencyclidine |
| 305.9 | – Abuse |
| 304.60 | – Dependence |
| 292.89 | – Intoxication |
| 292.9 | – Phencyclidine-Related Disorder NOS |
| 304.80 | Polysubstance Dependence |
| 309.81 | Posttraumatic Stress Disorder |
| ----- | Psychotic Disorder |
| 293.81 | – Due to...*[Indicate the General Medical Condition]*, With Delusions |
| 293.82 | – Due to...*[Indicate the General Medical Condition]*, With Hallucinations |
| 298.9 | – NOS |

**R**

313.89    Reactive Attachment Disorder of Infancy or Early Childhood
299.80    Rett's Disorder

**S**

295.70    Schizoaffective Disorder
-----         Schizophrenia
295.20         – Catatonic Type
295.10         – Disorganized Type
295.30         – Paranoid Type
295.60         – Residual Type
295.90         – Undifferentiated Type
295.40    Schizophreniform Disorder
-----         Sedative, Hypnotic, or Anxiolytic
305.40         – Abuse
304.10         – Dependence
292.89         – Intoxication
292            – Withdrawal
313.23    Selective Mutism
309.21    Separation Anxiety Disorder
300.23    Social Phobia
300.81    Somatization Disorder
300.82    Somatoform Disorder NOS
300.29    Specific Phobia

**T**

307.20    Tic Disorder NOS
307.23    Tourette's Disorder
307.21    Transient Tic Disorder

# Appendix E:
# Suggested Rating Scales

Rating scales can be helpful screening tools during the evaluation process or to monitor treatment progress. As opposed to providing an exhaustive list of all rating scales, suggested rating scales have been chosen. The selection criteria for these scales include those that are relatively easy to complete, provide reliable and valid information, align well with assessment or treatment monitoring goals, are primarily patient and/or parent report, and can be easily scored by support staff.

Please note that there are many useful scales beyond those that are listed. Inclusion of any scale does not imply an endorsement by the authors as a better scale nor does exclusion of any scale imply that it is less useful. The selected scales are ones that the authors are comfortable using and reflect their own preferences.

Ordering information is provided for scales that are copyrighted, web links are provided for those that are public domain or free, and a reference is provided when online sources are not available. This list does not include neuropsychological assessments or educational assessments. The focus is on rating scales that can be administered, scored, and interpreted in a pediatrician's or PCP's office.

## General Screening

*Child Behavior Check List (CBCL)*: This is a commonly used general assessment. It is designed for children and adolescents between 1.5 to 18 years of age. There is a preschool form for children between 1.5 and 5 as well as a general form for youths between 6 and 18. Each of these has approximately 110 items. It is also known as the "Achenbach."
Internet: www.aseba.org

*Pediatric Symptom Checklist (PSC)*: This is a 35-item scale used commonly in pediatric and primary care settings. It is primarily used for children and adolescents between 6 and 16 years of age, but can be applied to children as young as 4. It is available in English, Spanish, and Japanese.
Internet: http://psc.partners.org

## ADHD

*Vanderbilt ADHD Diagnostic Parent Rating Scale*: This approximately 50-item scale is available as a parent and a teacher report. It is used for children and adolescents between the ages of 6 and 12.
Internet: www.brightfutures.org

*Connors Rating Scales – Revised*: This approximately 75-item scale is for youths between ages 3 and 17. It includes a parent report and a teacher report, as well as an adolescent self-report.
Internet: www.pearsonassessments.com

## Anger

*State-Trait Anger Expression Inventory (STAXI)*: This 44-item scale is designed to measure adolescents' perceptions of anger as either a situationally bound emotion (state) or a characteristic of self (trait). It also measures control and expression of anger. T scores are displayed for 6 subscales; scores from 60 to 69 indicate a mild level of clinical elevation; scores of 70 or above are considered to be clinically elevated. Subscales include state anger, angry temperament, anger held in, anger control, trait anger, angry reaction, anger expressed, and anger expression frequency.
Internet: www.parinc.com

*Children's Inventory of Anger (CHIA)*: This 39-item scale for children and adolescents between ages 6 and 16 identifies situations that provoke anger in particular children, as well as the intensity of their anger response. T scores in the range of 50 to 59 are considered mild clinical elevation; scores of 60 and above are considered clinically elevated. Subscales include frustration, physiological, peer, and authority.
Internet: http://portal.wpspublish.com

## Anxiety Symptoms

*Multidimensional Anxiety Scale for Children (MASC) – Short Version*: This 14-item scale consists of 10-items designed to measure symptoms of anxiety. It is used for youths between the ages of 8 and 19. T scores from 60 to 70 indicate a mild level of clinical elevation; scores of 70 or above are to be considered clinically elevated.
Internet: www.mhs.com

*Self-Report for Childhood Anxiety Related Emotion Disorders (SCARED)*: This 41-item scale is used with children and adolescents aged 8 and above. Scores greater than 25 suggest the presence of an anxiety disorder and scores greater than 30 are considered more specific. It assesses for general anxiety, panic disorder or somatic symptoms, generalized anxiety disorder, separation anxiety disorder, social anxiety disorder, or significant school avoidance.
Internet: http://www.wpic.pitt.edu/research/

*Yale-Brown Obsessive Compulsive Scale (Y-BOCS)*: This 20-item scale is used with youths aged 14 and above. There is also a child version (CY-BOCS), which has 40 items and is used with children between 6 and 14 years. Both versions are clinician administered.
Internet (Y-BOCS): http://www.brainphysics.com/research/ybocs.pdf
Reference (CY-BOCS): Scahill L, Riddle MA, McSwiggen-Hardin M, et al. Children's Yale-Brown Obsessive Compulsive Scale: reliability and validity. *J Am Acad Child Adolesc Psychiatr*. 1997;*36*(6):844-52.

## Depression Symptoms

*Reynolds Adolescent Depression Scale (RAD-2)*: This 30-item scale is used with youths between 11 and 20 years of age. There is a child version, the Reynolds Child Depression Scale (RCDS), for children between the ages of 8 and 12 years. A T score and a percentile score are generated for comparison to age norms. A T score of 61 is consistent with clinical depression, with scores of 61–64 indicating mild symptoms, 65–69 for moderate symptoms, and 70+ for severe symptoms.
Internet: www.parinc.com

*Children's Depression Inventory (CDI)*: This 27-item scale is used with children and adolescents between 7 and 17 years of age. It helps to assess cognitive, affective, and behavioral signs of depression. T scores that are 65 and above are considered clinically elevated. Subscales include negative mood, interpersonal difficulties, negative self-esteem, ineffectiveness, and anhedonia.
Internet: http://www.pearsonassessments.com/tests/cdi.htm

## Suicide

*Suicide Probability Scale (SPS)*: This 36-item scale is used with youths aged 14 and above. It produces 4 subscale T scores that are summed to find a total score. Subscales include hopelessness, suicide ideation, negative self evaluation, and hostility. T scores from 60 to 69 indicate a mild level of clinical elevation. T scores of 70 and above should be considered clinically elevated.
Internet: http://portal.wpspublish.com

## Trauma

*Trauma Symptom Checklist for Children (TSCC)*: This 54-item scale for children and adolescents between the ages of 8 and 16 measures trauma-related symptomatology. It generates 10 subscale T scores for specific symptoms as well as under-reporting and hyper-reporting scales, which indicate the validity of the self-report: T scores from 60 to 69 indicate a mild level of clinical elevation; scores of 70 or above are considered clinically elevated. Subscales include under-report, depression, dissociation, sexual concerns, hyper-report, anger, dissociation-overt, sexual preoccupation, anxiety, PTSD, dissociation-fantasy, and sexual distress.
Internet: www.parinc.com

## Self-Perception

*Harter Self-Perception Profile (HARTER)*: This instrument contains 45 items and 9 subscales. It is designed for children and adolescents over the age of 8 and evaluates self-perception along specific domains. The highest mean score is 4.0. A lower mean score implies lower self-esteem in that domain. Subscales include social acceptance, physical appearance, close friendships, athletic competence, romantic appeal, behavioral conduct, scholastic competence, global self-worth, and job competence.
Reference: Harter S. *The Self-Perception Profile for Children: Revision of the Perceived Competence Scale for Children*. Denver: University of Denver; 1985.

# Appendix F:
# References and Sources for Additional Information

American Academy of Child and Adolescent Psychiatry. Practice parameters for the assessment and treatment of children and adolescents with anxiety disorders. *J Am Acad Child Adolesc Psychiatr*. 2007;46(2):267-283.

American Academy of Child and Adolescent Psychiatry. Practice parameters for the assessment and treatment of children and adolescents with attention-deficit/hyperactivity disorder. *J Am Acad Child Adolesc Psychiatr*. (in press).

American Academy of Child and Adolescent Psychiatry. Practice Parameters for the Assessment and Treatment of Children and Adolescents with Bipolar Disorders. *J Am Acad Child Adolesc Psychiatr*. 2007;46(1):107-125.

American Academy of Child and Adolescent Psychiatry. Practice parameters for the assessment and treatment of children and adolescents with oppositional defiant disorder. *J Am Acad Child Adolesc Psychiatr*. 2007;46(1):126-141.

American Academy of Child and Adolescent Psychiatry. Practice parameters for the assessment and treatment of children and adolescents with substance use disorders. *J Am Acad Child Adolesc Psychiatr*. 2005;44(1):1-25.

American Academy of Child and Adolescent Psychiatry. Practice parameters for the assessment and treatment of children and adolescents with reactive attachment disorder of infancy and early childhood. *J Am Acad Child Adolesc Psychiatr*. 2005;44:1206-1219.

American Academy of Child and Adolescent Psychiatry. Practice parameters for the assessment and treatment of children and adolescents with schizophrenia. *J Am Acad Child and Adolesc Psychiatry*. 2001;40(7 Suppl):4S-23S.

American Academy of Child and Adolescent Psychiatry. Practice parameters for the assessment and treatment of children and adolescents with suicidal behavior. *J Am Acad Child Adolesc Psychiatr*. 2001;40(7 Suppl): 24S-51S.

American Academy of Child and Adolescent Psychiatry. Practice parameters for the assessment and treatment of children, adolescents, and adults with autism and other pervasive developmental disorders.

*J Am Acad Child Adolesc Psychiatr*. 1999;38(12 Suppl):32S-54S.

American Academy of Child and Adolescent Psychiatry. Practice parameters for the assessment and treatment of children, adolescents, and adults with mental retardation and comorbid mental disorders. *J Am Acad Child Adolesc Psychiatr*. 1999;38(12 Suppl):5S-31S.

American Academy of Child and Adolescent Psychiatry. Practice parameters for the assessment and treatment of children and adolescents with depressive disorders. *J Am Acad Child Adolesc Psychiatr*. 1998;37(10 Suppl):63S-83S.

American Academy of Child and Adolescent Psychiatry. Practice parameters for the assessment and treatment of children and adolescents with language and learning disorders. *J Am Acad Child Adolesc Psychiatr*. 1998;37(10 Suppl):46S-62S.

American Academy of Child and Adolescent Psychiatry. Practice parameters for the assessment and treatment of children and adolescents with obsessive-compulsive disorders. *J Am Acad Child Adolesc Psychiatr*. 1998;37(10 Suppl):27S-45S.

American Academy of Child and Adolescent Psychiatry. Practice parameters for the assessment and treatment of children and adolescents with posttraumatic stress disorder. *J Am Acad Child Adolesc Psychiatr*. 1998;37(10 Suppl):4S-26S.

American Academy of Child and Adolescent Psychiatry Official Action. Practice parameters for the assessment and treatment of children and adolescents with anxiety disorders. *J Am Acad Child Adolesc Psychiatr*. 1997;36(10 Suppl):69S-84S.

American Academy of Child and Adolescent Psychiatry. Practice parameters for the assessment and treatment of children and adolescents with bipolar disorder. *J Am Acad Child Adolesc Psychiatr*. 1997;36(10 Suppl):157S-176S.

American Academy of Child and Adolescent Psychiatry. Practice parameters for the assessment and treatment of children and adolescents with conduct disorder. *J Am Acad Child Adolesc Psychiatr*. 1997;36(1):1-42.

American Academy of Child and Adolescent Psychiatry. Practice parameters for the assessment and treatment of children and adolescents with conduct disorder. *J Am Acad Child Adolesc Psychiatr*. 1997;36(10 suppl):122S-139S.

American Academy of Child and Adolescent Psychiatry. Practice parameters for the psychiatric assessment of children and adolescents. *J Am Acad Child Adolesc Psychiatr*. 1997;36(10 suppl):4S-20S.

American Academy of Child and Adolescent Psychiatry. Practice parameters for the assessment and treatment of children, adolescents and adults with attention-deficit/hyperactivity disorder. *J Am Acad Child Adolesc Psychiatr*. 1997;36(10 suppl):85S121S.

American Academy of Child and Adolescent Psychiatry. Practice parameters for the assessment and treatment of children and adolescents with substance use disorders. *J Am Acad Child Adolesc Psychiatr*. 1997;36(10 suppl):140S-156S.

American Academy of Child and Adolescent Psychiatry. Practice parameters for the psychiatric assessment of infants and toddlers (0–36 months). *J Am Acad Child Adolesc Psychiatr*. 1997;36(10 suppl):21S-36S.

American Academy of Child and Adolescent Psychiatry. Practice parameters for the psychiatric assessment of children and adolescents. *J Am Acad Child Adolesc Psychiatr*. 1996;34:1386-1402.

American Academy of Child and Adolescent Psychiatry Committee on Mental Retardation and Developmental Disabilities. The roles and responsibilities of child and adolescent psychiatry in the field of developmental disabilities. *Am Acad Child Adolesc Psychiatry News*. 1998 Winter;7.

American Academy of Pediatrics. Clinical practice guideline: Treatment of the school-aged child with attention deficit/hyperactivity disorder. *Pediatrics*. 2001;108:1033-144.

American Academy of Pediatrics Committee on Quality Improvement, Subcommittee on Attention-Deficit/Hyperactivity Disorder Clinical Practice Guideline. Diagnosis and evaluation of the child with attention-deficit/hyperactivity disorder. *Pediatrics*. 2000;105(5):1158-1170.

American Psychiatric Association. Practice guideline for the treatment of patients with acute stress disorder and posttraumatic stress disorder. *Am J of Psychiatry*. 2004;(7):1-57.

American Psychiatric Association. *Diagnostic and Statistical Manual of Mental Disorders*. 4th ed. (text rev.). Washington, DC: American Psychiatric Association; 2001.

Angold A, Costello EJ. Toward establishing an empirical basis for the diagnosis of oppositional defi-

ant disorder. *J Am Acad Child Adolesc Psychiatr*. 1996;35:1205-1212.

Barbaresi WJ, Katusic SK, Colligan RC, et al. How common is attention deficit/hyperactivity disorder? *Arch Pediatr Adolesc Med*. 2002;15:217-224.

Barkley RA. Psychosocial treatments for attention-deficit hyperactivity disorder in children. *J Clin Psychiatry*. 2002;63(Suppl 12):36-43.

Barkley RA. *Taking Charge of ADHD: The Complete, Authoritative Guide for Parents*. New York: Guilford; 1996.

Barkley RA. *Attention-Deficit Hyperactivity Disorder: A Handbook for Diagnosis and Treatment*. 2nd ed. New York, Guilford; 1998.

Barkley RA. *Defiant Children: A Clinician's Manual for Assessment and Parent Training*. 2nd ed. New York: Guilford Press; 1997.

Barret PM, Duffy AL, Dadds MR, et al. Cognitive-behavioral treatment of anxiety disorders in children: long-term (6-year) follow-up. *J Consult Clin Psychol*. 2001;69:135-141.

Bashe PR, Kirby BL. *The Oasis Guide to Asperger's Syndrome*. New York: Crown; 2001.

Bauer M. *Field Guide to Psychiatric Assessment and Treatment*. Philadelphia: Lipponcott Williams & Wilkins; 2003.

Beitchman JH, Young A. Learning disorders with a special emphasis on reading disorders: a review of the past 10 years. *J Am Acad Child Adolesc Psychiatr*. 1997;36:1020-1032.

Bernstein GA, Layne AE, Egan EA, et al. School-based intervention for anxious children. *J Am Acad Child Adolesc Psychiatr*. 2005;44:1118-1127.

Biederman J, Hirshchfeld-Becker DR, Rosenbaum JF, et al.. Further evidence of association between behavioral inhibition and social anxiety in children. *Am J Psychiatry*. 2001;158:1673-1679.

Biederman J, Wilens T, Mick E. Is ADHD a risk factor for psychoactive substance use disorders? Findings from a four-year prospective follow-up study. *J Am Acad Child Adolesc Psychiatr*. 1997;36:21-29.

Biederman J, Faraone SV, Marrs A, et al. Panic disorder and agoraphobia in consecutively referred children and adolescents. *J Am Acad Child Adolesc Psychiatr*. 1997;36:214-223.

Biederman J, Faraone S, Milberger S, et al. A prospective 4-year follow-up study of attention-deficit hyperactivity and related disorders. *Arch Gen Psychiatr*. 1996;53:437-446.

Birmaher B, Khetarpal S, Brent D, et al. The Screen for Child Anxiety Related Emotional Disorders (SCARED): scale construction and psychometric characteristics. *J Am Acad Child Adolesc Psychiatr.* 1997;36:545-553.

Black B, Uhde TW. Treatment of elective mutism with fluoxetine: a double blind placebo-controlled study. *J Am Acad Child Adolesc Psychiatr.* 1994;33:1000-1006.

Boris NW, Dalton R, Forman MA. Mood disorders. In: Behrman RE, Kliegman RM, Jenson RB, eds. *Nelson Textbook of Pediatrics.* 17th ed. Philadelphia: Saunders; 2004.

Briere J, Johnson K, Bissada A, et al. The Trauma Symptoms Checklist for Young Children: reliability and association with abuse exposure in a multisite study. *Child Abuse Negl.* 2001;25:1001-1014.

Brown RT, Amler RW, Freeman WS et al. Treatment of attention-deficit hyperactivity disorder: Overview of the evidence. *Pediatrics.* 2005;115(6):e749-e757.

Brown RL, Henke A, Greenhalg H, et al. The use of haloperidol in the agitated, critically ill pediatric patient with burns. *J Burn Care Rehabil.* 1996;17:34-8.

Burke JD, Loeber R, Birmaher B. Oppositional defiant disorder and conduct disorder: a review of the past 10 years, part II. *J Am Acad Child Adolesc Psychiatr.* 2002;41:1275-1293.

Burns DD. *Feeling Good: The New Mood Therapy.* New York: William Morrow and Company; 1980.

Calhoun J. Classroom Modification of Elective Mutism. *Behav Therapy.* 1973;4:700-702.

Campbell M, Adams PB, Small AM, et al. Lithium in hospitalized aggressive children with conduct disorder: a double-blind and placebo-controlled study. *J Am Acad Child Adolesc Psychiatr.* 1995;34:445-453.

Cepeda C. Concise Guide to the Psychiatric Interview of Children and Adolescents. Washington, DC: American Psychiatric Press Inc; 2000.

Carskadon MA, Dement WC. Daytime sleepiness: quantification of a behavioral state. *Neurosci Biobehav Rev.* 1987;11:307-317.

Cheng K, Myers KM. *Child and Adolescent Psychiatry: The Essentials.* Philadelphia: Lippincott Williams & Wilkins; 2005.

Cheng-Shannon, J., McGough, J.J., Pataki, C. et al. Second-generation antipsychotic medications in children and adolescents. *J Child Adol Psychopharmacol.* 2004;14(3):372-394.

Clarke GN, Rohde P, Lewinsohn PM, et al. Cognitive behavioral group treatment of adolescent depression: efficacy of acute treatment and booster sessions. *J Am Acad Child Adolesc Psychiatr.* 1999;38:272-279.

Correll, C.U., Leucht, S., Kane, J.M. Lower risk for tardive dyskinesia associated with second-generation antipsychotics: A systematic review of 1-year studies. *Am J Psychiatry.* 2004;161:414-425.

Costello EJ, Pine DS, Hammen C, et al. Development and natural history of mood disorders: advances. *Child Adolesc Psychiatr Clin N Am.* 2000;9:159-182.

Culpepper, L. Use of algorithms to treat anxiety in primary care. *J Clin Psychiatry.* 2003;64(Suppl 2):30-33.

Davis, LL, Ryan, W, Adinoff, B, et al. Comprehensive review of the psychiatric uses of valproate. *J Clin Psychopharmacol.* 2000;20(1)(Suppl 1):1S-17S.

DelBello M, Greevich S. Phenomenology and epidemiology of childhood psychiatric disorders that may necessitate treatment with atypical antipsychotics. *J Clin Psychiat.* 2004;65(Suppl 6):12-19.

Dias PJ. Adolescent substance abuse assessment in the office. *Pediatr Clin N Am.* 2002;49:269-300.

Donnelly CL, Amaya-Jackson L, March JS. Psychopharmacology of pediatric posttraumatic stress disorder. *J Child Adolesc Psychopharmacol.* 1999;9:203-220.

Dow, SP, Sonies BC, Scheib D, et al. Practical guidelines for the assessment and treatment of selective mutism. *J Am Acad Child Adolesc Psychiatr.* 1995;4:836-846.

Dulcan MK, ed. *Helping Parents, Youth, and Teachers Understand Medications for Behavioral and Emotional Problems: A Resource Book of Medication Information Handouts.* 3rd ed. Washington DC: American Psychiatric Publishing Inc; 2006.

Dummitt ES III, et al. Systematic assessment of 50 children with selective mutism. *J Am Acad Child Adolesc Psychiatr.* 1997;36:653-660.

Dummit ES III, et al. Fluoxetine treatment of children with selective mutism: an open trial. *J Am Acad Child Adolesc Psychiatr.* 1996;35:615-621.

Duncan M, Martini D, Lake M. *Concise Guide to Child and Adolescent Psychiatry.* 3rd ed. Washington, DC: American Psychiatric Publishing Inc; 2003.

Emslie GJ, Ryan ND, Wagner KD. Major depressive disorder in children and adolescents: Clinical trial design and antidepressant efficacy. *J Clin Psychiatry.* 2005;66(Suppl 7):14-20.

Expert Consensus Guideline Series. Optimizing pharmacologic treatment of psychotic disorders. *J Clin Psychiatry.* 2003;64(Suppl 12):1-100.

Fassler DG, Dumas LS. *Help Me I'm Sad: Recognizing, Treating, and Preventing Childhood and Adolescent Depression.* New York: Viking; 1997.

Ferber, R. *Solve Your Child's Sleep Problems*. New York: Fireside; 2006.

Findling RL, Steiner H, Weller FB. Use of antipsychotics in children and adolescents. *J Clin Psychiatry*. 2005;66(Suppl 17):29-40.

Findling RL. Treatment of aggression in children: Primary care companion, *J Clin Psychiatry*. 2003;5(Suppl 6):5-9.

Fosnocht KM, Ende J. Approach to the patient with fatigue. *UpToDate Online*, version 15.1; 2006.

Francis PD. Effects of psychotropic medications on the pediatric electrocardiogram and recommendations for monitoring. *Curr Opin Pediatr*. 2002;14:224-230.

Fremont WP. School refusal in children and adolescents. *Am Fam Physician*. 2003;68(8):1555-64.

Fristad MA, Goldberg Arnold JS. *Raising a Moody Child: How to Cope with Depression and Bipolar Disorder*. New York: Guilford Press; 2004.

Gargus RA, Yatchmink Y. Early Identification and assessment of young children with autism. *Med Health*. 2005;88(5):147-151.

Geller B, DelBello MP, eds. *Bipolar Disorder in Childhood and Early Adolescence*. New York: Guilford Press; 2003.

Geller B, Zimerman B, William M, et al. Phenomenology of prepubertal and early adolescent bipolar disorders: examples of elated mood, grandiose behaviors, decreased need for sleep, racing thoughts and hypersexuality. *J Child Adolesc Psychopharmacol*. 2002;12:3-9.

Geller B, Zimerman B, William M, et al. DSM-IV mania symptoms in a prepubertal and early adolescent bipolar disorder phenotype compared to attention-deficit hyperactive and normal controls. *J Child Adolesc Psychopharmacol*. 2002;12:11-25.

Gerdtz J, Bregman J. *Autism: A Practical Guide for Those who Help Others*. New York: Continuum; 1990.

Gibson AP, Bettinger, TL, Patel, NC, et al. Atomoxetine versus stimulants for treatment of attention deficit/hyperactivity disorder. *Ann Pharmacother*. 2006;40(6):1134-1142.

Goddard, A.W., Shekhar, A., Anand A. et al. Psychopharmacology of pediatric anxiety disorders. *Int Drug Ther Newsl*. 2002;37(12):89-94.

Greene RW. *The Explosive Child*. New York: Harper Paperbacks; 2005.

Green WH. *Child and Adolescent Clinical Psychopharmacology*. 4th ed. New York: Lippincott Williams & Wilkins; 2007.

Grundy SM, Cleeman JI, Daniels SR, et al. Diagnosis and management of the metabolic syndrome: an American Heart Association/National Heart, Lung, and Blood Institute scientific statement. *Circulation*. 2005;112:2735-2752.

Hayward C, Killen JD, Taylor CB. Panic attacks in young adolescents. *Am J Psychiatry*. 1989;146:1061-1062.

Henggeler SW, Clingempeel WG, Brondino MJ, et al. Four-year follow-up of multisystemic therapy with substance-abusing and substance-dependent juvenile offenders. *J Am Acad Child Adolesc Psychiatr*. 2002;41:868-874.

Henggeler SW, Phillippe B, Cunningham SG, et al. Multisystemic therapy: an effective violence prevention approach for serious juvenile offenders. *J Adolesc*. 1996;19(1):47-61.

Howard BJ, Wong J. Sleep disorders. *Pediatr Rev*. 2001;22:327-342.

Hughes CW, Emslie GJ, Crimson ML, et al. The Texas children's medication algorithm project: report of the Texas consensus conference panel of medication treatment of childhood major depressive disorder. *J Am Acad Child Adolesc Psychiatr*. 1999;38(11):1442-1454.

Jellinek M, Patel BP, Froehle MC, eds. *Bright Futures in Practice: Mental Health-Volume I. Practice Guide*. Arlington, CA: National Center for Education in Maternal and Child Health; 2002.

Jellinek M, Patel BP, Froehle MC, eds. *Bright Futures in Practice: Mental Health-Volume II. Tool Kit*. Arlington, CA: National Center for Education in Maternal and Child Health; 2002.

Jellinek, MS, Snyder JB. Depression and suicide in children and adolescents. *Pediatr Rev*. 1998;19:255.

Kaminer Y, Jellinek S. Contingency management reinforcement procedures for adolescent substance abuse. *J Am Acad Child Adolesc Psychiatr*. 2000;39:1324-1326.

Kazdin, A, Weiss J. eds. *Evidence-based Psychotherapies for Children and Adolescents*. New York: Guilford Press; 2003.

Kearney CA. Dealing with school refusal behavior. A primer for family physicians: workable solutions for unhappy youth and frustrated parents. *J Fam Pract*. 2006;55(8):685-692.

Kearney CA, Albano AM. *Therapist's Guide for the Prospective Treatment of School Refusal Behavior*. San Antonio, TX: The Psychological Corporation; 2000.

Kearney CA, Albano AM. *When Children Refuse School: A Cognitive-Behavioral Therapy Approach*

*– Parent Workbook*. San Antonio, TX: The Psychological Corporation; 2000.

Kearney CA, Albano AM. *Therapist's Guide for the Prospective Treatment of School Refusal Behavior*. San Antonio, TX: The Psychological Corporation; 2000.

Kendall PC, Hedtke KA. *Cognitive-Behavioral Therapy for Anxious Children: Therapist Manual*. 3rd ed. Ardmore, PA: Workbook Publishing; 2006.

Kendall PC, Hedtke KA. *Coping Cat Workbook*. 2nd ed. Ardmore, PA: Workbook Publishing; 2006.

Kendall PC. Treating anxiety disorders in children: results of a randomized clinical trial. *J Consult Clin Psychol*. 1994;62:100-110.

Kim WJ, Enzer N, Bechtold D, et al. *Meeting the Mental Health Needs of Children and Adolescents: Addressing the Problems of Access to Care*. Washington, DC: American Academy of Child and Adolescent Psychiatry; 2001.

King BH, State MW, Shah B, et al. Mental retardation: a review of the past 10 years: part I. *J Am Acad Child Adolesc Psychiatr*. 1997;36:1656-1663.

Knight JR, Sherritt L, Shrier, et al. Validity of the CRAFFT substance abuse screening test among adolescent clinic patients. *Arch Pediatr Adolesc Med*. 2002;156(6):607-614.

Koplewicz H. *More Than Moody: Recognizing and Treating Adolescent Depression*. New York: G.P. Putnam's Sons; 2002.

Kotagal S, Pianosi P. Sleep disorders in children and adolescents. *Br Med J*. 2006;332:828-832.

Kovacs M. The Children's Depression Inventory (CDI). *Psychopharmacol Bull*. 1985;21:1995-998.

Labellarte MJ, Ginsburg GS, Walkup, JT, et al. The treatment of anxiety disorders in children and adolescents. *Biol Psychiatr*. 1999;46(11):1567-1578.

Leckman JF, Cohen DJ. *Tourette's Syndrome – Tics, Obsessions, Compulsions: Developmental Psychopathology and Clinical Care*. New York: Wiley; 2001.

Lewinsohn PM, Klein DN, Seeley JR. Bipolar disorders in a community sample of older adolescents: prevalence, phenomenology, comorbidity, and course. *J Am Acad Child Adolesc Psychiatr*. 1995; 34:454-463.

Lewinsohn PM, Clarke GN, Seeley JR, et al. Major depression in community adolescents: age at onset, episode duration, and time to recurrence. *J Am Acad Child Adolesc Psychiatr*. 1994;33:809-818.

Linehan MM, Heard HL, Armstrong HE. Naturalistic followup of a behavioral treatment for chronically parasuicidal borderline patients. *Arch Gen Psychiatr*. 1993;50:971-974.

Loeber R, Burke JD, Lahey BB, et al. Oppositional defiant and conduct disorder: a review of the past 10 years, part I. *J Am Acad Child Adolesc Psychiatr*. 2000;39:1468-1484.

Lyons MJ, True WR, Eisen SA, et al. Differential heritability of adult and juvenile antisocial traits. *Arch Gen Psychiatr*. 1995; 52:906-915.

Mammel K. Depression. In: Berman S, ed. *Pediatric Decision Making*. 4th ed. Philadelphia: Mosby; 2003.

Mammel K. Substance Abuse. In: Berman S, ed. *Pediatric Decision Making*. 4th ed. Philadelphia: Mosby; 2003.

Mancuso CE, Tanzi MG, Gabay M. Paradoxical reactions to benzodiazepines: Literature review and treatment options. *Pharmacotherapy*. 2004;24(9):1177-1185.

March JS, Parker JD, Sullivan K, et al. The Multidimensional Anxiety Scale for Children (MASC): factor structure, reliability, and validity. *J Am Acad Child Adolesc Psychiatr*. 1997;36:554-565.

March JS, Leonard HL, Swedo SE. Neuropsychiatry of obsessive-compulsive disorder in children and adolescents. *Compr Ther*. 1995;21:507-512.

Marcus MD, Kalarchian MA. Binge eating in children and adolescents. *Int J Eat Disord*. 2003;34:S47-57.

Martin A, Scahill L, Charney DS, Leckman JF, eds. *Pediatric Psychopharmacology*. New York: Oxford University Press; 2003.

Martin A, Volkmar FR, Lewis M, eds. *Child and Adolescent Psychiatry: A Comprehensive Textbook*. 4th ed. Philadelphia: Lippincott, Williams & Wilkins; 2007.

McClellan J, Werry J. Evidence-based treatments in child and adolescent psychiatry: an inventory. *J Am Acad Child Adolesc Psychiatr*. 2003;42(12):1388-1400.

McCloskey LA, Walker M. Posttraumatic stress in children exposed to family violence and single-event trauma. *J Am Acad Child Adolesc Psychiatr*. 2000;39:108-115.

McHolm AE, Cunningham CE, Vanier MK. *Helping Your Child With Selective Mutism*. Oakland, CA: New Harbinger Publications; 2005.

McKenna K, Gordon CT, Lenane M, et al. Looking for childhood-onset schizophrenia: the first 71 cases screened. *J Am Acad Child Adolesc Psychiatr*. 1994;33:636-644.

Mehler P. Diagnosis and care of patients with anorexia nervosa in primary care settings. *Ann Intern Med*. 2001;134:1048-1059.

Micromedex Healthcare Series (1974–2007). Thompson Healthcare, Inc.

Millman R. Excessive sleepiness in adolescents and young adults: causes, consequences, and treatment strategies. *Pediatrics*. 2005;115(6):1774-1786.

Miller CK, et al. An interdisciplinary team approach to the management of pediatric feeding and swallowing disorders. *Child Health Care*. 2001;30(3):201-218.

Mindell J, Owens J. *A Clinical Guide to Pediatric Sleep – Diagnosis and Management of Sleep Problems*. Philadelphia: Lippincott Williams and Wilkins; 2003.

Mufson L, Weissman MM, Moreau D, et al. Efficacy of interpersonal psychotherapy for depressed adolescents. *Arch Gen Psychiatr*. 1999;56:573-579.

Mufson L, Moreau D, Weissman MM, et al. *Interpersonal Psychotherapy for Depressed Adolescents*. New York: Guilford; 1993.

Newcorn JH, Strain J. Adjustment disorder in children and adolescents. *J Am Acad Child Adolesc Psychiatr*. 1992;31:318-326.

Nicholls D, Viner R. Eating disorders and weight problems. *Brit Med J*. 2005;330(7497):950-953.

Owens JA. Sleep disorders. In: Behrman RE, Kliegman RM, Jenson RB, eds. *Nelson Textbook of Pediatrics*. 17th ed. Philadelphia: Saunders; 2004.

Palla B, Litt IF. Medical complications of eating disorders in adolescents. *Pediatrics*. 1988;81:613-623.

Pavuluri MN, Birmaher B, Naylor MW. Pediatric bipolar disorder: a review of the past 10 years. *J Am Acad Child Adolesc Psychiatr*. 2005;44:846-871.

Pavuluri MN, Naylor MW, Janicak PG. Recognition and treatment of pediatric bipolar disorder. *Contemporary Psychiatry*. 2002;1(1):1-9.

Rapoport JL, Ismond DR. *DSM-IV Training Guide for Diagnosis of Childhood Disorders*. New York: Brunner/Mazel; 1996.

Rapopart JL. *The Boy Who Couldn't Stop Washing: The Experience and Treatment of Obsessive-Compulsive Disorder*. New York: Penguin; 1990.

Research Units on Pediatric Psychopharmacology Anxiety Study Group. The Pediatric Anxiety Rating Scale (PARS): development and psychometric properties. *J Am Acad Child Adolesc Psychiatr*. 2002;41:1061-1069.

Rynn MA, Siqueland L, Rickets K. Placebo-controlled trial of sertraline in the treatment of children with generalized anxiety disorder. *Am J Psychiatry*. 2001;158:2008-2014.

Sachs GS. Decision tree for the treatment of bipolar disorder. *J Clin Psychiatr*. 2003;64(Suppl 8):35-40.

Scahill L, Chappell P, Kim YS, et al. A placebo-controlled study of guanfacine in the treatment of children with tic disorders and attention deficit hyperactivity disorder. *Am J Psychiatr*. 2001;158:1067-1074.

Scahill L, Riddle M, McSwiggen-Hardin M, et al. Children's Yale-Brown Obsessive Compulsive Scale: reliability and validity. *J Am Acad Child Adolesc Psychiatr*. 1997;36:844-852.

Schwartz RH. Selective Mutism: Are Primary Care Physicians Missing the Silence? *Clin Pediatr*. 2006;45(1):43-48.

Shaffer D, Gould MS, Brasic J, et al. A Children's Global Assessment Scale (CGAS). *Arch Gen Psychiatr*. 1983;40:1228-1231.

Shaw RJ, DeMaso DR. *Clinical Manual of Pediatric Psychosomatic Medicine: Mental Health Consultation with Physically Ill Children and Adolescents*. Washington DC: American Psychiatric Publishing Inc; 2006.

Siegel B. *Help children with Autism Learn: A Guide to Treatment Approaches for Parents and Teachers*. Oxford: Oxford University Press; 2003.

Sigman GS. Eating disorders in children and adolescents. *Pediatr Clin N Am*. 2003;50(5):1139-1177.

Slattery MG, Bernstein GA. Anxiety disorders. In: Berman S, ed. *Pediatric Decision Making*. 4th ed. Philadelphia: Mosby; 2003.

Stahl SM, Grady MM, eds. *Essential Psychopharmacology: The Prescriber's Guide*. Cambridge, UK: Cambridge University Press; 2004.

State MW, King BH, Dykens E. Mental retardation: a review of the past 10 years: Part II. *J Am Acad Child Adolesc Psychiatr*. 1997;36:1664-1671.

Stein, MT, et.al. Selective mutism. *Pediatrics*. 2001;107:926-929.

Stein, MT, et.al. Two-year-old boy with language regression and unusual social interactions. *Pediatrics*. 2001;107:910-915.

Strober M, Carlson G. Bipolar illness in adolescents with major depression: clinical, genetic, and psychopharmacologic investigation. *Arch Gen Psychiatr*. 1982;39:549-555.

Stubbe D. *Child and adolescent psychiatry: A practical guide*. Philadelphia: Lippincott Williams & Wilkins; 2007.

Suppes T, Dennehy EB, Swann AC, et al. Report of the Texas Consensus Conference Panel on medication treatment of bipolar disorder 2000. *J Clin Psychiatr*. 2002;63(4):288-299.

Swedo SE, Leonard HL, Garvey M, et al. Pediatric autoimmune neuropsychiatric disorders associated with streptococcal infections (PANDAS): clinical description of the first fifty cases. *Am J Psychiatry*. 1998;155:264-271.

Swedo SE, Rapoport JL, Leonard H, et al. Obsessive-compulsive disorder in children and adolescents: clinical phenomenology of 70 consecutive cases. *Arch Gen Psychiatr*. 1989;46:335-341.

TADS Team. Treatment for Adolescents with Depression Study (TADS): rationale, design, and methods. *J Am Acad Child Adolesc Psychiatr*. 2003;42:531-542.

Tarter RE. Evaluation and treatment of adolescent substance abuse: a decision tree method. *Am J Drug Alcohol Abuse*. 1990;16:1-46.

Tourette's Syndrome Study Group. Treatment of ADHD in children with tics: a randomized controlled trial. *Neurology*. 2002;58:527-536.

Treatment for Adolescents With Depression Study Team. Fluoxetine, cognitive-behavioral therapy, and their combination for adolescents with depression: Treatment for adolescents with depression study (TADS) randomized controlled trial. *JAMA*. 2004;292:807-820.

Tuchman RF, et.al. Regression in pervasive developmental disorders: seizures and epileptiform electroencepphalogram correlates. *Pediatrics*. 1997;99:560-566.

Turkel SB, Taveré CJ. Delirium in children and adolescents. *J Neuropsychiatry Clin Neurosci*. 2003;15:431:435.

Van Gelder DW, Kennedy L, et.al. Congenital and infantile aphasia. *Pediatrics*. 1952;9(1):48-54.

Wagner KD. Diagnosis and treatment of bipolar disorder in children and adolescents. *J Clin Psychiatr*. 2004;65(Suppl 15):30-35.

Walkup JT, Labellarte MJ, Riddle MA, et al. Fluvoxamine for the treatment of anxiety disorders in children and adolescents. *N Engl J Med*. 2001;344:1279-1285.

Webster-Stratton C, Hammond M. Treating children with early-onset conduct problems: a comparison of child and parent training interventions. *J Consult Clin Psychol*. 1997;65:93-109.

Weinberg NZ, Rahdert E, Colliver JD, et al. Adolescent substance abuse: a review of the past 10 years. *J Am Acad Child Adolesc Psychiatr*. 1998;37:252-261.

Weston JA. Growth deficiency/failure to thrive. In: Berman S, ed. *Pediatric Decision Making*. 3rd ed. St. Louis: Mosby; 1996.

White T, Anjum A, Charles Schulz SC. The Schizophrenia prodrome. *Am J Psychiatr*. 2006;163:376-380

Wiener JM, Dulcan MK, eds. *Textbook of Child and Adolescent Psychiatry*. 3rd ed. Washington, DC: American Psychiatric Press Inc; 2003.

Wilkes TCR, Belsher G, Rush AJ, et al. *Cognitive Therapy for Depressed Adolescents*. New York: Guilford; 1994.

Wills L, Reiff MI. Sleep disturbances. In: Berman S, ed. *Pediatric Decision Making*. 4th ed. Philadelphia: Mosby; 2003.

Wise MG, Brandt G. Delirium. In: Hales RE, Yudofsky SC, eds. *Textbook of Neuropsychiatry*. 2nd ed. Washington DC: American Psychiatric Press Inc; 1992.

Wozniak J. Recognizing and managing bipolar disorder in children. *J Clin Psychiatr*. 2005;66(Suppl 1):18-23.

Youngstrom EA, Findling RL, Calabrese JR, et al. Comparing the diagnostic accuracy of six potential screening instruments for bipolar disorder in youth aged 5 to 17 years. *J Am Acad Child Adolesc Psychiatr*. 2004;43:847-858.

Younus M, Labellarte MJ. Insomnia in children: When are hypnotics indicated? *Pediatr Drugs*. 2002;4(6):391-403.

## Additional Helpful Websites

Academy of Cognitive Therapy
www.academyofct.org

American Academy of Child and Adolescent Psychiatry
www.aacap.org

American Academy of Pediatrics
www.aap.org

American Psychiatric Association
www.psych.org

Child and Adolescent Bipolar Foundation
www.bpkids.org

Children and Adults with Attention Deficit Hyperactivity Disorder (CHADD). www.chadd.org.

Federation of Families for Children's Mental Health
www.ffcmh.org

National Alliance for the Mentally Ill (NAMI)
www.nami.org

National Center for Learning Disabilities
www.ncld.org

National Institute on Drug Abuse (NIDA)
www.nida.nih.gov

National Institute of Mental Health
www.nimh.nih.gov

Parents Medication Guide
www.parentsmedguide.com/

Surgeon General's Report on Mental Health
www.surgeongeneral.gov/library/mentalhealth

Substance Abuse and Mental Health Services Administration
www.samhsa.gov

*Kalyna Z. Bezchlibnyk-Butler, Adil S. Virani (Editors)*

# Clinical Handbook of Psychotropic Drugs for Children and Adolescents

2nd, revised and expanded edition 2007, 348 pages
spiral-bound, US $62.00 / € 49.95, ISBN: 978-0-88937-309-9

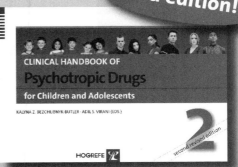

## A new edition of the highly acclaimed psychotropic drug reference for all clinicians dealing with children and adolescents!

This book is designed to fill a need for a comprehensive but compact and easy-to-use reference for all mental health professionals dealing with children and adolescents. The new edition of the widely praised handbook summarizes the latest information from the published literature (scientific data, controlled clinical trials, case reports) and clinical experience in compact and easy-to-use charts and bulleted lists for each class of psychotropic drug used in children and adolescents.

The spiralbound handbook includes for each class of drugs both monograph statements on use in children and adolescents and approved indications, as well as the available data concerning off-label indications, findings from open and double-blind studies concerning doses, adverse effects, and other considerations in these age groups.

For each class of drug, summary information is provided on: Classification • Product availability • Indications • Pharmacology • Dosing • Pharmacokinetics • Adverse effects • Withdrawal • Precautions • Toxicity • Nursing implications • Drug interactions • Contraindications • Patient instructions • Interactions

### From the reviews of the first edition:

*"Authoritatively and exhaustively compiles currently available information in a user-friendly form... The aim of the Handbook is to be a source of 'fast facts' for the busy clinician... an aim it achieves splendidly."* M. Gittelman, *Int J Mental Health*, 2005

*"Well-researched... An essential reference book... Full of indispensable information and data in a sequenced and logical design."* P. Shelley, *Drogo Res – Int J Psychiatric Nursing Res*, 2004

*"Provides the busy clinician with all the information that is essential for those prescribing a psychotropic drug to a child or adolescent... Very 'user friendly'... Highly recommended to all clinicians that specialize in treating children and adolescents."* B.E. Leonard, *Human Psychopharmacol*, 2005

*"If you see children who are placed on psychotropic medications, this books clearly falls into your 'must-have' category."* J.C. Courtney, *Child Neuropsychol*, 2005

### Table of Contents

Order online at: **www.hogrefe.com** or call toll-free **(800) 228-3749**

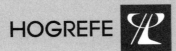

Hogrefe Publishing · 30 Amberwood Parkway · Ashland, OH 44805
Tel: (800) 228 3749 · Fax: (419) 281 6883 · E-Mail: custserv@hogrefe.com
Hogrefe Publishing · Rohnsweg 25 · 37085 Göttingen, Germany
Tel: +49 551 999 500 · Fax: +49 551 999 50 425 · E-Mail: custserv@hogrefe.de

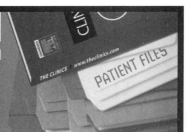
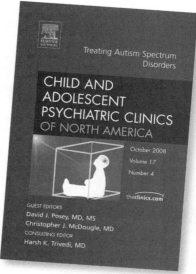
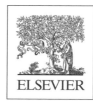